Letters from the Clinic

In every field of therapeutic practice a significant amount of time is spent writing letters about and to patients. In *Letters from the Clinic* Derek Steinberg applies detailed literary and psychological analysis to over forty letters, highlighting why certain words or phrases were used, how they could have been put better, and builds around them principles and theoretical positions based on narrative therapy, consultative approaches and the psychological impact of words and phrases.

Using the context of child, adolescent and family psychiatry, while also applicable to all therapeutic work, the book deals with issues such as

- explaining terminology, clinical conditions and treatments
- the second opinion
- confirming clinical contracts
- conveying difficult advice and painful news
- confidentiality and consent
- everyday practical matters – appointments, maintaining contact, billing, informal messages
- what patients think of letters.

Each letter is accompanied by detailed annotations and discussion.

Letters from the Clinic will prove a valuable tool to all those working in clinical and therapeutic practice.

Derek Steinberg is a Consultant in Child and Adolescent Psychiatry. He trained in Oxford, at the Maudsley and at the Tavistock Institute in London. He worked at the Maudsley and Bethlem Royal Hospitals where he directed the Adolescent Unit for twenty years before going on to Ticehurst House Hospital in Sussex. He has published six books and taught widely in the UK and abroad, and has a special interest in the relationships between literature and the arts and psychiatry.

Letters from the Clinic

Letter writing in clinical practice
for mental health professionals

Derek Steinberg

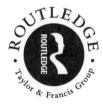

London and Philadelphia

First published 2000 by Routledge
11 New Fetter Lane, London EC4P 4EE

Simultaneously published in the USA and Canada
by Taylor & Francis Inc
325 Chestnut Street, 8th Floor, Philadelphia PA 19106

Routledge is an imprint of the Taylor & Francis Group

Typeset in Times by Keystroke, Jacaranda Lodge, Wolverhampton
Printed and bound in Great Britain by Biddles Ltd, Guidlford and King's Lynn

British Library Cataloguing in Publication Data
A catalogue record for this book is available from the British Library

Library of Congress Cataloging in Publication Data
Steinberg, Derek.
    Letters from the clinic : letter writing in clinical practice for mental health
professionals / Derek Steinberg.
        p. ; cm.
    Includes bibliographical references and indexes.
    1. Child psychotherapy. 2. Letter writing–Therapeutic use. I. Title: Letter
writing in clinical practice for mental health professionals. II. Title.
    [DNLM: 1. Child Psychiatry–methods. 2. Correspondence. 3. Adolescent
Psychiatry–methods. WS 350 S819L 2000]
    RC489.W75 S74 2000
    618.92'89165–dc21   00–024896

ISBN 0–415–20503–4 (hbk)
ISBN 0–415–20504–2 (pbk)

Contents

Foreword

Many clinicians including, I regret to admit, myself have regarded letters as a necessary but largely irrelevant distraction from the main business of the clinical treatment of patients. What Steinberg does in this book is to get us to bring the letter into the main frame of our clinical work. He shows us that this is important, that it is as much part of the clinical treatment of a patient as anything else we do.

There is a very long tradition of doctor writers. Some like Chekhov or Conan Doyle used their talents away from medicine. Others have used their interest and ability to write in the furtherance of their main profession through research or teaching. Steinberg is one of this kind and has written extensively on a wide range of subjects within his speciality. He is thus an experienced clinician and a writer. He has an interest in the written word and how it affects those who read it. He knows that for patients who come to possess our written words as something independent from the clinical encounter there is a kind of separateness or distance of the subject from the clinician. He knows how the written word can be valuable in a rather special way but also how it can be a problem, sometimes even dangerous, when taken out of context and misunderstandings cannot be corrected as they can in a face-to-face meeting.

What is interesting and quite unique about this book is that we do not simply have a good writer using his talent to communicate professional knowledge, we have a medical writer, a word-smith using his dual crafts to help us. We all have to be medical writers even though most of us are not very good ones. We often deal with this by concentrating on what we do well and what interests us and neglect this whole section of our professional lives and, by that useful defence of denial, fail to notice how our letters affect our patients and our colleagues often in ways that would shock us if only we knew it. Steinberg helps us to be sensitive to our patients' experiences when they receive our letters. When we know this we can use our letters to help our patients to prepare themselves, to upset or even traumatise them less. By turning his attention to this whole area of clinical practice Steinberg not only helps us rescue a neglected area but also really extend our clinical effectiveness. He shows us that we have a powerful clinical tool which we can use as a real adjunct to our usual 'in the consulting room' clinical practice. Many of us have a long way to go and it does take practice to develop letter-writing skills but Steinberg gives us a great deal of help and shows us, with his often beautiful examples, how we can do it. Some of his best examples are quite short. The carefully thought-out wording, careful explanations of what we need to say, the consideration of whom we write to, what we call them and what we call ourselves, can enhance rather than as so often happens complicate and hamper our work.

Reading this book is like having a series of very valuable tutorials which can make a real difference to the quality of clinical practice.

Robin Anderson
Consultant Psychiatrist and Chairman of the
Adolescent Department, Tavistock Clinic
January 2000

Preface

The letters in this book are all made up. They are genuine enough nonetheless; every phrase or line used to make a point having been taken from a real letter from the files, and the matters they illustrate cover a wide range of the practical problems that come up every day in clinical and therapeutic work with young people and their families. It is a complex field, and diagnosis and treatment rarely get far without touching on (or stumbling into) quite problematic issues of categorisation, confidentiality, ethics, legality, and interdisciplinary work and relationships. Characteristically the work demands practical and sometimes urgent action, yet it is full of the ambiguities and uncertainties that make such action difficult (Eisenberg, 1975). There is something about the extra care demanded of work with children and adolescents, amplified by the related fact that so much of it is necessarily under cross-disciplinary and public scrutiny, and the fact that adolescents are old enough to be noisily articulate about problems but too young to be 'grown-up' about them, which makes this a demanding, turbulent and rather raw subject. I believe these same characteristics mean that what child and adolescent psychiatry and related work have to handle today, many other areas of medical, psychological and social work will have to face tomorrow, so that the sorts of matters these letters illustrate will be found to have a wider relevance outside psychiatry.

Confidentiality and consent are two such areas, and of course I have gone to great lengths to make sure that real people's cases, and indeed the professionals involved, cannot be identified. Obviously, all the names and locations are fictitious, and if the kaleidoscopic process of juggling names and situations appears to present the image of a case you think you know, then that can only be one of those unavoidable coincidences.

The primary point of this book is the power of words and the value of choosing them thoughtfully in the fields referred to above. This is self-evident in psychotherapy, but it is at least as important in that broadly psychotherapeutic penumbra around all clinical work. I have tried to make the theme of each letter sufficiently interesting to render the business of finding the right words worthwhile; meanwhile the process of finding the right words illuminates the theme from a different angle from that of the textbook. I hope this reciprocity makes letter writing an interesting exercise as well as a learning tool; but it is the process of trying to say the right thing that I want to convey, not the end result as such; hence, this isn't intended to be a handbook of model letters.

Whom and what to acknowledge? We all send, read and receive acres of letters, and it's amazing that there is so little teaching on them. I have been guided, informed and misinformed by thousands over the years; good letters, bad letters and indifferent letters, and some so awful – some by me – they make the hair stand on end. One experience that drew them to my attention was a tradition in the professorial unit at the Maudsley Hospital where a group of registrars would be required to read to each other the letters they had written that week, and not, as would firmly be pointed out, for the purposes of mutual congratulation.

I also want to acknowledge the Tavistock Clinic and Institute, every bit as critical and hard-headed as the Maudsley, though less overtly macho about it, and in particular the consultation training programme and a series of associated seminars in which I participated, led by Dorothy Heard, Irene Caspari, Denise Taylor and John Bowlby. Consultation has grown out of Gerald Caplan's original work (1970) as an adaptable and multi-purpose tool, yet with some quite precise rules (Steinberg, 1989, 1993). It is ideally suited to many contemporary problems in the organisation and use of health services, and I have tried to translate some of its philosophy and practice into guiding principles when writing clinical letters.

The third influence I want to acknowledge is simply that broad and growing stream of psychotherapeutic and family therapeutic work that has become steadily less rigid and ideologically bound in recent years, and more pragmatic and human as it has matured and its practitioners have grown in confidence. As it has developed it has leaned towards clarification and away from mystification and become more compatible with consultative approaches, with each learning from the other. There is a direct link between what I learned with my colleagues during twenty years at the Maudsley's Adolescent Unit at Bethlem Royal Hospital, and what has gone, suitably transformed and disguised, into the letters in this book.

Much is owed, also, to teaching in which I have been involved over the years, when I have used art and writing techniques to work with groups on team development and service organisation issues. Whether in this country or abroad, the themes that emerged were very much the same, and the process of finding the right words and phrases to identify group and team processes was also similar, with or without the help of translators. Indeed, I have often been struck by the self-deception and illusion involved when people believe they speak the same language. Finding the right word was sometimes a more precise and productive exercise when participants *didn't* formally speak the same language, because the nature of the task became more obvious. I would particularly like to acknowledge Dr Jack Hung, Rachel Poon and their colleagues at the Child, Adolescent and Family Clinic, Kowloon, Hong Kong; Giorgios Polos of the Arts and Therapy Centre and the Adolescent Day Hospital in Athens; Dr Danai Papadatou of the Faculty of Nursing, the University of Athens; Professor Andrzej Rajewski of the Academy of Medicine, Poznan; Dr Irena Namyslowska, Head of the Department of Child and Adolescent Psychiatry, in the Warsaw Institute of Psychiatry; Professor Jaczek Bomba of the

Faculty of Medicine of the Jiagellonian University, Cracow; the staff of the De Beele Clinic, Voorst, Holland; Miss Ang Bee Lian of the Ministry of Community Development, Singapore; Christiane Francois of the British Council, Port of Spain, and the sixth formers of the Trinidad and Tobago schools who took part in the careers workshop I attended there; Professor Shozo Aoki of Kawasaki Medical School for his advice and help with my Clinical Letters workshop there; and, in the UK, Dr Sourangshou Acharyya, Dr Roland Littlewood, Lennox Thomas, Chriso Andreou, Mona Wilson and, with sadness, the late Dr Jafar Kareem of NAFSIYAT, the Inter-Cultural Therapy Centre in London, all of whom in various ways enabled, encouraged and helped with a wide range of opportunities, exercises and experiments, all to do, in the end, with finding the right word; Dr David Goldberg for his inspiring teaching on emplotment in clinical letters; Dr Spiros Karvounis, with whom I worked in a series of psychotherapy seminars at Ticehurst House Hospital, and for whom tracking down the origins of words and meanings is a hobby, an academic pursuit and an obligation; and finally, in the task of ending up with the right words on paper, I am indebted to Ann King, Copy Editor, for her many useful suggestions and eagle-eyed attention to detail.

Mentioning the Maudsley, the Tavistock and Ticehurst among other exotic places is a reminder about another aspect of confidentiality, a necessarily recurring theme in this book: that it is far easier to disguise a patient than an institution, and that institutions can be vulnerable to what is said or inferred about them, whether justified or not. The clinical and training experiences on which the letters that follow are based are made up from correspondence, notes and recollections drawn quite randomly and from a very wide field, in the UK and elsewhere, well beyond the above three institutions, and so imply nothing in particular about them. The letters are perhaps best regarded as documentary fiction.

The letters which were the focus of the survey reported in Chapter 9, however, were real, and were written from the Young People's Unit at Ticehurst House Hospital. I am grateful to Dr Herb Etkin, Director of the Unit and Medical Director of the hospital, Margaret Cudmore, General Manager, and to the hospital's Ethics Committee for giving permission for the study, to the family doctors and families who returned the questionnaires, and to Jennifer Steward and Christine Gramstadt for their respective work in co-ordinating the survey and assessing the results.

Much of this book consists of letters and numbered notes on the letters followed by some general comments. I have covered a fairly wide range of clinical and related themes to illustrate various points, but the book is far from comprehensive. However, as many clinical conditions and events are mentioned, I have added a separate clinical index to the general one in case some readers should find the book useful as an introduction to child and family psychiatry, albeit via an unusual route.

Two practical points. First, the points indicated thus[1] in the letters aren't always in numerical order; nor are they followed in precisely the same order in the notes that follow, because the flow of the comments doesn't always match the order

Chapter 1

Introduction
Reasons for writing

Why write?

First, because finding the right words is a good exercise, and committing them to paper adds to the responsibility to get it right; when you get it wrong it will in due course stare you in the face without the option of retrospective falsification or fudge about what you believed you made clear. So putting it in writing self-critically is good practice, whatever the reason for doing so.

Second, and to turn to the most important reason as far as this book is concerned, because of the importance of words in therapy; any therapy, not just psychotherapy. The right words capture or convey a feeling or an attitude in a way that contributes to the therapeutic process, just as the wrong words can undermine it. This applies as much to the clinical relationship in general (for example, a surgeon explaining about an operation, or a physician advising about medication) as it does to psychodynamic psychotherapy; arguably more so, because in the latter there is more going on and over a longer period, and there is a dynamic, too, in getting it right, and in the therapist finding out what getting it right is going to entail. The clinician hoping to be therapeutic outside the quite tight rules and regime of formal psychotherapy might have only one opportunity, even an unanticipated one, to capture the clinical moment helpfully in the right words. It is this, sometimes transient, even fleeting opportunity in general clinical work that can be grasped and used therapeutically; an extreme example might be saying goodbye helpfully to an angrily departing patient. When writing it down – authoritatively, thus assuming responsibility as its *author* – we take quite a chance, not least because the words can be reread, for example, in moments when the patient, not the therapist, is managing the *Gestalt* – the whole picture.

The ability to find the right word is a clinical and therapeutic skill and, like all such skills, can be developed. What is needed is to be truthful without being hurtful, discourteous or undermining therapy. One should avoid jargon – but what *is* jargon? Some dictionary definitions describe it as specialised language, in which case it is not only discourteous but inefficient to use it in attempts at communication with a non-specialist audience. (On the subject of words I would say *communication* is a good example of a word borrowed from ordinary language for use as jargon, and is now half-way back into everyday language to identify something with which many people are preoccupied these days; so where does that leave it?) Other definitions give pretentiousness as a characteristic of jargon, which implies flawed communication, because if a word is used to demonstrate how much more the speaker or writer knows than the reader, the word is falling short in its prime purpose of conveying meaning. My impression is that most users of jargon intend neither to impress nor confuse, but simply forget that useful technical shorthand within a specialised group can be meaningless and apparently pretentious outside it. But ignorance is no excuse. I suppose jargon becomes psychobabble (itself jargon) when psychological concepts are used to impress, divert, confuse, or amaze; or as a form of surfing, the speaker or babbler jumping euphorically from technical term to technical term too fast for the listener to grasp (or criticise) either the general drift or the precise meaning of each word. None the less we all have our preferences, and one person's plain English might seem like jargon to another. Some people whose care with language I respect are baffled by my own dislike of 'ongoing' and 'meaningful', words which I will take great detours to avoid, and scratch out aggressively when entrusted with editing. Political correctness is a grisly area too, and one which I will try to tackle later.

Using euphemistic words and phrases is another tricky area; no doubt many examples are to be found in this book. One might report, for example, that what Mr X says he did is quite different from what he said last week, or how others regularly describe his behaviour, all of which is a little on the weaselly side; or one might say Mr X is a liar. The latter may help the exasperated observer to feel better, but the former construction is more likely to provide something to work on. Nor is it necessarily less accurate.

Then there is the simpler matter – simpler conceptually, but every bit as difficult linguistically – of speaking your mind in a direct and spontaneous way and contributing helpfully at the same time. Much is made of speaking one's mind, indeed as if it is a moral duty, though it is quite possible to speak one's mind and still talk nonsense.

A third reason for writing is because a letter can take the form of an agreed treatment plan, an *aide-mémoire*, an informal contract between therapist, patient and family, and the beginnings of an agenda for the next meeting. It thus provides affirmation of what has happened so far, the opportunity to reconsider or challenge what has been set down as 'agreed', as well as continuity. Life goes on in the 167 hours or more between, say, weekly sessions, and the letter, even if it is only vaguely recalled rather than a constant source of interest, can help keep up the momentum of treatment. Writing it down reveals fudges or ambiguities which need clarifying, though ambiguity can be useful (see p. 117); thus an ambiguity stated clearly in writing can be a useful launching pad to dealing with it. Another advantage of a letter is that it can refer to or be addressed to people who can help but who weren't present at the session.

Fourth, there is magic in the written or spoken word; this is discussed below.

Even modern, computer-printed prescription forms sometimes begin with the magic symbol Rx,[1] though I believe it is more potent when handwritten.

Fifth, everyone has a right to know what is being said or written about them in a potentially public (i.e. shared) document, although I believe that this needs to be set against another right: that of keeping one's own personal thoughts in note form. However, this too has been disputed, on the grounds that if a professional thought X at a particular time, even if it was written only in his or her private diary (e.g. 'check dose of Z'), in some circumstances this could be of wider significance.

Sixth, moral and ethical issues apart, patients do have an increasing right to see their own notes (Bernadt *et al.*, 1991; Brahams, 1994; Gauthier, 1999; McLaren, 1991; Parrott *et al.*, 1988) and are increasingly likely to exercise it. Why not write *all* notes in the expectation that, at some point, they may be read? Writing letters is good practice for this.

Seventh, because every sort of professional worker can learn from other experts' and specialists' letters. General practitioners sometimes point out how useful a contribution to postgraduate training a good letter from a specialist can be. Might clear, jargon-free letters about problems, aims and methods present the 'psycho-social' professions and our clientele in a more positive light?

Finally, although careful writing can be time-consuming, it speeds up with practice, and in any case pausing to think about our clientele and their problems does us and them no harm, and letter writing provides a framework for this. A steady improvement in the ratio of thinking time to writing time should be anticipated, with both steadily diminishing, and writing notes and dictating letters might become less of a chore and even interesting. If writing notes is boring, we may be writing the wrong sort of notes.

A study of psychiatrists' letters to general practitioners showed that the writing improved after the introduction of a departmental auditing procedure focusing on guidelines for letter writing; this followed the implementation of the 1990 Access to Health Records Act (Shah and Pullen, 1995). It seemed there was less use of jargon, value judgements and pejorative remarks following the audit, though the amount of information in the letters remained the same and they were of much the same length.

Auditing procedures can be perceived as intrusive and even threatening, but if conducted sensibly, by which I would mean in a consultative rather than supervisory way, they can make a valuable contribution to peer–peer teaching. One of the attractions of the consultative approach is its reciprocity: peer–peer discussion of a problem or piece of work along consultative lines is also, by definition – i.e. in the very nature of consultation – a learning exercise, while conversely, a learning or audit exercise can be built on consultative discussion of a piece of work (Steinberg, 1989, 1993). Letter writing is ideal as a focus for such teaching.

---

1 Rx is the symbol for Jupiter, or Jove, under whose special protection those who take medicines are placed. The symbol is shorthand for the following injunction: 'Under the good auspices of Jove, the patron of medicines, take the following drug in the prescription laid down.'

What do the recipients of letters think?

Thus the writing of such letters is a very good thing. But what do their recipients think? Curiously enough little seems to have been reported about this, particularly in psychiatry (Pierides, 1999). It is discussed in Chapter 9.

The magic of words

It comes as something of a surprise to discover that *glamour* means spelling. The word, which in modern usage conveys all sorts of wonder, splendour, authority and prestige, both spurious and real, derives from the words *grimoire* and *grammaire*, twelfth- or thirteenth-century Old French for a book of spells. Thus glamour means grammar, and this means getting the words right if you want the spell (or prescription) to work, which after all is largely what this book is about.

While playing with words, an activity I want to encourage, the relationship between *author* and *authority* is interesting, though perhaps not immediately obvious. The pathway from an author's mind through the marks he or she makes on paper to the images they create in the reader's head represents a most extra-ordinary alchemy, in whatever detail we try to track the sociocultural, technical and neural pathways for the process. It takes an extraordinary sort of authority, and acceptance of that authority, for a fiction writer to establish, often in the first few phrases, interest, curiosity and even concern about a character or situation woven in only a handful of tiny printed squiggles. Many such characters are more real to us than historical figures, although the latter have also benefited significantly from the attentions of writers of fantasy and fiction, and still do. A large literature has grown up which relates narrative – fact or fiction – to psychological development at every level, from the sociocultural to the personal. The writing of letters is not part of narrative psychology, but there are important areas of overlap, where the patient's tale, so to speak (and indeed the wife's tale, and the daughter's tale, and the general practitioner's tale, and so on), is compared on paper with the therapist's tale. It is therefore worth looking briefly at some of the concepts of narrative – story-telling – in relation to psychotherapy.

Narrative and mythology

Myths are cultural stories which provide a background, frame of reference and therefore guide to how life is to be handled and how decisions are to be made; for example, such basic things as what is 'good' or 'bad', acceptable or unacceptable. The word 'myth' is often used disparagingly, for example, in dismissing classical psychoanalytical writings as merely mythology, yet myths are powerfully influential, and we should be interested in such powerful influences on human psychology. Civilisations rise and fall on the backs of myths, and it seems inherently unlikely that major wars would start without a foundation in mythology; indeed, military strategists talk of the importance of generating a 'war psychosis' as soon as politicians think a war is needed, so that the appropriate stories can begin to be told. Thus myths may not always be nice, but they are very powerful (can they be more destructive than nuclear weapons?) and should not be underestimated at any level of human activity (Steinberg, in press).

Myths are not all bad. We need them anyway, like food, and they can supply the essential, the nutritious, the non-nutritious and the frankly poisonous. Campbell (1973) provides a monumental account of the place of myths in human culture, poetically describing myths as public dreams, and dreams as private myths. Bettelheim's *The Uses of Enchantment* (1976) describes how fairy-tales help children to grow up, and Dwivedi and Gardner (1997) describe story-making in terms of developmental psychology and therapy, namely as an activity central to organising and structuring experience.

Narrative as clinical history

Traditionally, the clinician 'takes a history'; in other words, he or she writes the patient's story. It is likely to be part fact, part fiction, part autobiography, part biography, and in any case partial. The clinician is likely to be guided by the story he or she likes to write (for example, about psychoneurology, developmental psychology, social relationships or psychoanalysis); the eclectic practitioner writes a book of short stories. We cannot help being influenced by the conceptual models in our heads (Tyrer and Steinberg, 1998) and, while it is right to strive to be objective (including being objective about our subjective impressions, if we can), on philosophical or neuropsychological grounds it seems inherently unlikely that we can be completely objective. Many psychotherapists of course are less inclined to 'take (i.e. write) a history', and more inclined to simply let the client talk and thus assume responsibility and authority for his or her own story.

It does seem likely, on the face of it, that people have more than one story to tell, all different and all true. Individual lives and relationships are immensely complex, and what is remembered at any given time, or given significance at any given time, and the ambiguities and range of both feelings and thoughts about these kaleidoscopic experiences, are likely to produce a subtly or grossly different tale depending on the time and circumstance in which it is requested. It will also vary according to state of mind; brain chemistry and structural change, with or without effects on memory, will profoundly influence the story. It will also be affected by what the speaker makes of the listener, and what he or she wants the other person to hear. Finally, of course, all these influences on the clinical interview are no more than a sample of the influences of daily life, which proceeds within a matrix of self-image and the perceptions and expectations of others. Thus whatever else is going on in terms of neurochemistry or social change, the individual is perpetually trying and sometimes failing to piece it all together, adding, editing, filling and making gaps, in a continuous process of attempting to make sense of it all, and in a way which underpins consciousness and psychological existence. I take it that it isn't controversial to describe one strand of human development in this way.

But, to move from the individual to the family model, the individual as auto-biographical writer is not alone in his or her task. Relatives and acquaintances are busily writing too, producing scripts for (for example) the teenager as failure, or as success and scholar, for the good mother, the bad father, the efficient sibling and so on.

The narrative perspective of the client's history is that he or she may need editorial help; thus: the therapist as editor. (Even, in the case of a *really* odd manuscript, a good agent?)

Narrative in therapy

Dwivedi and Gardner (1997), Frank (1993), Roberts and Holmes (1999) and White and Epston (1990) provide excellent and comprehensive reviews of the relationships between story-telling, psychological development and therapy, with the individual's development of a personal mythology (and the power of other people's attributed mythologies) as common themes. Another important theme is the role of the narrative in providing distance between the individual and a painful event (for example, bereavement or other trauma), yet without compromising involvement (Ayalon, 1990; Shiryon, 1978), the story thus acting as a medium for creating both enough involvement and distance for the necessary work to be done in terms of personal development or therapeutic work. 'Distancing' in terms of story-telling is understandable enough as a powerful device, even bordering, constructively, on denial (as when an injured or abused child is helped to talk about what happened to Teddy), but conversely the powerful capacity of reading, and imagination generally, to involve a child should not be underestimated. Winnicott (1972) has discussed the importance, as a process but also as an indicator of maturation, for the child to be securely 'alone' and lost in play, a phenomenon which Nell (1988) relates to people of all age groups in their experience of reading: 'lost in a book'. He quotes Gass' poetic words (1972) that 'it seems incredible, the ease with which we sink through books quite out of sight, pass clamorous pages into soundless dreams.' Holmes (1994) and Roberts and Holmes (1999) relate the experience of being *able* to be lost in this way – i.e. it is a strength and a capacity – to the attachment theory dynamic for there being someone *holding* the individual child (or vulnerable person of any age) securely enough in the personal environment for such exploration to be feasible. At another level the spellbinding story-teller does the same.

Can a letter achieve this? No doubt some can, but the sorts of everyday letters described in this book, largely to do with the initiation and maintenance of clinical engagement rather than psychotherapy, borrow from concepts of narrative therapy rather than represent it. In an equivalent way I would say that much in traditional psychotherapy and cognitive behaviour therapy uses, or is illuminated by, notions of narrative therapy: as aphorisms, vignettes or self-contained and focused episodes, rather than the full story.

White and Epston (1990) give a comprehensive account of the use of narratives in therapy, and in which they include letter writing and 'certification', that is, giving an individual who has made an achievement a document or declaration to that effect. They construct their approach around the political philosophy of Michel Foucault, which is essentially about the hidden power in social institutions and groups to affect members of those groups, something which Foucault has expounded upon in a particular way (e.g. Foucault, 1980), linking it to the need for comprehensive revolution (e.g. a new form of proletarian justice which does without a judiciary). Unless I have missed something, I am not convinced that White and Epston's adaptation of Foucault to therapy does more than point out that individuals can be trapped in power structures that include their own and others' knowledge (ideas, assumptions, attributions) as an integral part, and that the point of therapy is to enable them to see this and adopt alternatives. What this leads to, however, is the use of what they term *externalisation*, that is, externalisation of the problem, thereby giving the 'victim' (to stay with the model for the moment) the opportunity, authority and vantage point to look at the problem from outside and join in the process of deciding who is doing what to whom. Thus the patient sees the story and has the opportunity to rewrite it. Using the concepts of psychodrama and role play, I would say that the patient is reminded, or informed, that he or she has a part in a play, and they might like to help rewrite the script, the description of their role and the way the performance is being directed.

Whatever the process of stepping out of the frame, one way of doing so is by writing. The authors provide a valid enough model, but I would place Foucault, despite his distinction as a political philosopher, simply among the many other theorists and practitioners who, so to speak, discovered 'society' (and prototype societies like groups and families) as somewhere to look for sources of distress and disability other than inside the patient's head. What I find more helpful than the political psychology of cultural power in White and Epston's account is the dynamics of the act of writing itself. Like Stubbs (1980), they hold that the use of writing in therapy legitimises and formalises *local popular knowledges* (his words, my italics), gives them continuity, and allows 'the independent authority of individuals, and the creation of a context for the emergence of new discoveries and possibilities'.

This, I believe, is potentially therapeutic, particularly the rather quaintly termed 'local popular knowledges'. This, to me, focuses on the truly local, the microcosm of the therapeutic dyad or group, with the assumption (that I would make, at least in child and adolescent psychiatry) that other people can be invited into that group (subpoenaed?), in role play or in imagination, to help take a look at the length, breadth and depth of 'the problem' and to formulate 'knowledge' which is indeed local and shared. Some of the letters in this book refer to examples of this. (But *does* it owe something to Foucault's notion of justice without a judiciary? Possibly, if the therapists take care not to be in that role themselves.)

The point is also made that writing illustrates events happening in sequence (an interesting contradistinction from, say, painting) which in turn can affirm the process of change in an individual's life, and thus the written tradition introduces the linear conception of time (White and Epston, 1990). We can therefore see the beginning of a usable dynamic between the open systems model of multiple mutual, reciprocal and to an extent circular effects (e.g. Bateson, 1972, 1979; Minuchin *et al.*, 1980; Von Bertalanffy, 1968), and the linear model used in common sense (A and B cause C), with the former model being used in therapy to see why the show has come off the road, and the latter to see it safely on its way again, with some written directions.

Letter writing in the context of narrative therapy

While sending letters isn't narrative therapy, the way in which letters are put together, and the way it is hoped they will be read, can benefit from this field. The abbreviation of White and Epston's account given above illustrates its connections with social constructionist theory (e.g. Berger and Luckmann, 1967; Hoffman, 1990) which is about our knowledge and our understanding of reality growing out of what we experience as individuals in relationships, groups and cultures. Take, for example, a gay person in a culture that regards homosexuality as an illness; in a culture that regards it as simply 'bad'; and in culture that perceives it as no less a part of the normal scene than, say, being male or female. How that person 'sees himself' or 'is seen' is not only a metaphor for how he *is* in each of these cultures, but, to be literal about it, how he might be written about, for example in personal correspondence, or in the newspapers. There are endless instances: the psychopath as wicked villain or as war hero, for example, again depends on how an individual's behaviour at a particular time in a particular context is perceived and, again, written about. In any therapy which adopts this biographical perspective, what the person assumes about himself or herself, and what others assume (homosexual, disabled, ill, disturbed, getting better) is regarded as having more in common with a novel, a not necessarily accurate biography, or, as mentioned above, a script, rather than as being 'objective fact'. As a piece of documentary fiction the text can be changed, in a process which Mattingly has described as therapeutic emplotment (1994). At its simplest it is, as already said, as if someone with a troubling self-image and pessimistic understanding of the future needs not so much a therapist as a new editor or director. On the one hand, the subject seems complex and radical, as something is bound to, which requires us to take a completely different perspective of reality. On the other hand, the traditional clinical approach is to *take the patient's history*, and then to write (prescribe) a script which may involve attending talking sessions in the role of client, going to the chemist's for a prescription, going into hospital or lying on an operating table – all of which constitute familar enough scenarios. Thus we use narratives anyway, in a constant dialogue with ourselves and others and about others; the challenge is in not only realising it, but in appreciating that rewriting is possible.

King *et al.* (1998) discuss the use of written assignments in therapy, a piece of work which gains from being slower and more thoughtful than most talking. They make the interesting point that people who are not used to writing things down may not have realised how the speaking voice differs from the written one. Penn and Frankfurt (1994) have described the value in terms of emotional change within and between family members when they write for each other. These approaches have been developed into what L'Abate and Platzmann (1991) have called programmed writing (PW) and which involves a wide range of tasks, such as keeping a diary or writing to and about themselves and each other.

That which makes narrative and in particular written forms of therapy useful has implications for letter writing, though for the purposes of this book the letter writing is in one direction only; *correspondence* as therapy would be a different subject, and an interesting one.

Writing it down is, for most people, different; it is slower; there is more to organise, whether it is a matter of loading another tape into the dictaphone, getting the word processor started, or organising one's thoughts.

Reflecting about what one is going to *say*, quite likely 'rewriting' as one goes along, is profoundly different from speech. There is a loss of spontaneity, if perhaps a gain in precision, but there might be disadvantages as well as advantages to both spontaneity and precision. Spontaneous speech is full of 'ers' and pauses and backtracking ('no, I mean . . . what do you call it . . . to put it another way') which would look and be different on paper. Yet the display of facial and body language and the vocal 'background music' accompanying the words contributes to the exchange of information in a variety of ways which include the positive, the negative, the clarifying and the confusing – probably all at the same time; and constantly monitored and modified by the other person's equally elaborate skills and performance. Writing it down is different, and there are both gains and losses.

It is also an intellectual exercise, unless the writer and the reader are proficient poets who *make* something (*poesis*) affective as well as cognitive of what is written. Of course feelings are communicated, but is the writer sure about what he or she wants to communicate? And does he or she succeed? Might it be successful one afternoon but not the following morning? Or would it have been more successful had the letter been read again, later, instead of being thrown away? For all the possibilities of achieving more focus and accuracy in writing than in speech, of generating particular sorts of feeling (intended or otherwise) and of dealing with issues, nevertheless, as Sloman and Pipitone (1991) point out, letter writing is a limited medium; it can be a means of avoiding confrontation, it is a distancing exercise and and one that displaces some of the necessary work.

For all its advantages, its limitations need to be borne in mind every time, literally or metaphorically, one puts pen to paper. As long as the difference is grasped, however, it can stand as a valuable distillation of aspects of the therapeutic process.

A note on political correctness

Political correctness (PC) is too large a subject for the purposes of this book, but I think it should be mentioned briefly, since the context here is the use of language.

The use of words and particularly forms of reference and address alter gradually with changes in the culture; for example, first names are more readily used as social roles and hierarchies become less rigid. There is a perspective, however, largely based on updated Marxist and social constructionist theory (see p.7), that any such changes are bound to operate slowly and in any case in the interests of those at the top of the hierarchy; so, rather than wait for social changes to influence the use of words, changes in such use should be imposed to alter the ways people think. This is precisely the process which George Orwell saw in his experience of socialist and national socialist tyrannies, and which he described in his dystopian work *Nineteen Eighty-four*, in which the state systematically tinkers with the language to produce *Newspeak*, a language in which certain words are no longer available and hence certain forms of thinking are no longer possible (Orwell, 1949; Young, 1991). In the imposition of PC thinking today the dictator of the prescribed language tends not to be the state directly, but the influence of the intellectual elite on the state.

Some may feel that this is how it should be. Where political correctness has been in step with cultural changes some good has come of it. To take one example: it is not right, still less accurate, to refer to successful professionals only as 'he', if anyone still does. The contortions of male authors in the prefaces to their books to explain their particular way of squaring this circle deserves a thesis. I think 'he or she' is best, with random use of 'he' or 'she' for variety, but I think 'he/she' is prissy and contrived. Correspondingly, if racially insulting language isn't inhibited by common kindness and courtesy, it seems to me right for the PC machinery to hoover it up.

Nevertheless, even if aspects of PC are no more than updated if enforced politenesses, and occasionally something to joke about, the means if not all the ends of PC are quite sinister. The problem comes back to the definition of the term. *'Politically correct'* derives directly from tyrannies where the elite political class knows best, certainly better than 'the masses'. The latter, until they have had their 'consciousnesses raised' (i.e. been re-educated), are encouraged to rely on their superiors' political analysis and not on their own traditional and therefore flawed common sense. Thus they do not have (or at least express) an opinion of their own, but, until or unless they acquire the skills, time and opportunity to learn the prescribed way of thinking, they must rely on the official *correct view*. They are otherwise deemed bad, mad or not properly educated. That is what political correctness means, and it isn't funny.

Writing is good for you

Although this book is about letters as a supplement to therapeutic work, rather than writing itself as therapy, Ellis' short paper (1989) on the therapeutic benefits for *patients* who write letters to their doctors (which he calls epistotherapy) makes a number of points which do have some relevance here. First, he describes letter writing as something for the patient to do, an emotional outlet which is immediately available and an occupier of mind and hand, and one which does not have a particular time limit, unlike the consultation. It also creates a degree of continuity outside the session when needed. Perhaps these things can sometimes benefit the therapist too?

For Ellis goes on to suggest more specific benefits for the doctor when writing to patients, relatives or colleagues, recommending explicit language (with expletives undeleted) and with as much venom as is felt necessary for the therapeutic effect. He then advises, 'file and wait for the healing process to take place'. This takes about a week. *Never* let anyone get hold of this file, Dr Ellis warns. If symptoms persist, the letters may then be sent, but with the expletives deleted. However, in his experience, rereading the unedited, unsent letters is usually sufficiently beneficial.

'Writing it down' in relation to the consultative model

Believing in the appropriateness of multiple conceptual models in clinical work, I think it is worth considering for a moment two of the great archetypal models of care: the *medical* and the *consultative*. The former is about expertise: the specialist, by virtue of his or her training, can *tell* (note the authority in the word) what is wrong with the individual and prescribes (writes down) the therapy that is most likely to help. I would maintain that this model, frequently criticised as representing typically medical authority, is in fact used regularly by psychologists and psychotherapists when they 'understand' their clients in terms (psychodynamic, behavioural, sociopolitical) rooted in training which the client hasn't had. It is a very good model for certain types of problem, but quite different from the *consultative* model, where the practitioner's skill is to do with restraining himself or herself and assisting clients to frame the problem and possible solutions in their own way. I have pointed out elsewhere (Steinberg, 1989) that while this approach to problem-solving has grown out of Caplan's work specifically on ways in which professional workers in various fields can operate together (e.g. Caplan, 1970), it has much in common with Carl Rogers' client-centred therapy (e.g. Rogers, 1951), in which, again, the skill lies in helping clients identify problems and solutions for themselves. (The fact that there is something of a category confusion here, in that consultation's strength is that it is not therapy, and Rogerian therapy's strength is that it is like consultation, should not divert us from the fact that here we have two rather similar ways of solving different types of problem.)

Having said which, I will now compound the matter by proposing that since both medical and consultative methods are useful we can employ both approaches, because it makes no sense for the therapist to be ideologically pure if the problems he or she sees are multifactorial. Since we have come thus far without saying what child and adolescent psychiatry is like, or at least how it appears to me, I will illustrate the point with a case vignette.

A 13-year-old boy is referred because of severely disabling obsessive-compulsive behaviour. This is a condition which has been much studied by psychologists and psychiatrists in recent years, its description usefully refined, and effective treatments developed. These include behaviour therapy and medication. The clinicians know what to advise, the boy's parents are appreciative, but the boy, though sometimes suicidal in his despair about his symptoms, is ambivalent. With the indecisiveness and anxiety for control characteristic of people with obsessional problems, while he makes it clear that he wants help, including the specific treatment offered, he constantly changes his mind about accepting it. On several occasions the parents have brought him back after an appointment, before even leaving the hospital grounds, because he has changed his mind, and this cycle of indecision goes on and on.

The clinical, legal and ethical issues are complex, but, for the sake of the point being made, it comes down to a conflict between several sorts of authority. There is the technical authority of the clinicians, who know what is needed as surely as anything is ever known in psychiatry and psychotherapy. The authority to accept treatment, however, rests uneasily between mother, father and teenager, with no decision being reachable, except, by default, the decision to procrastinate; but procrastination is part of the problem. One strategy, curiously one that is in keeping both with some versions of family therapy and with the worst of Victorian doctoring, would be to dismiss the patient and his parents until they come back with a sustainable decision. Another would be for the clinical team to force the issue (and impose treatment) in some way, perhaps resorting to legal steps to do so, something which is by no means invariably inappropriate, though it would be in this case.

Another way, and the one which illustrates the dual medical/consultative model I am recommending, is to openly acknowledge the problem of dispersed and different authority in the boy's case, so that the focus becomes a family therapeutic one: how, if and when to make a decision about the clinical expertise that is available. This approach doesn't render a difficult case easy, but it does clarify what is going on, who is responsible for what, and requires the clinicians *genuinely* to consult the boy and his parents about how to proceed. Letters were useful in a similar case (p. 5) which turned out quite well. Other, similar situations haven't.

To summarise, since whether to be prescriptive or consultative may depend more on the personality and ideology of the therapist than on the needs of the case, what is being suggested is a dual prescriptive/consultative model, in which, through what might be termed the primary consultation, an attempt is made to reach clarity and agreement about which problems are the responsibility of the clinician, and which the responsibility of the client.

This approach incorporates a fundamental tenet of consultative work: that all those involved are willing to learn from each other; thus the client finds out about what the therapist knows about 'this sort of case', which requires the clinician to do some teaching (and perhaps some reading), while the clinician learns, with genuine interest and curiosity, what the client's experience, feelings and views are. Whatever follows is likely to be based on properly informed consent (Steinberg, 1992a). This model is pursued throughout the letters that follow, and is the closest thing I have to an underlying principle or theory for them.

Some principles

1 A letter should reflect the clinical work to which it refers, by summing up work done thus far, not in general the writer's further reflections. So far we have identified letter writing with a broadly consultative approach; in other words, negotiations confirmed or continued in writing. Much therapeutic work is quite directive or instructive, and this is as true of individual, group and family therapeutic work as it is of the 'traditional' medical approach. Thus family therapists identify 'distortions', resistance to change and other devious processes in the family structure and apply strategies to change them (see e.g. Dare, 1985; Gorell Barnes, 1985, 1994), and most forms of psychotherapy, with the exception of Rogerian client-centred counselling (see p. 11), set out to do much the same. Curiously, in the light of the historical perceptions of the psychotherapies being supposedly rather 'open' and human, compared with behaviour therapy being mechanistic and authoritarian, it tends to be behaviour therapy as it is now practised which most requires the client to frame the problem, agree the way forward and monitor progress. It is not that therapeutic work should not be directive, rather that the style of some clinical work appears to be non-directive (e.g. the use of paradoxical injunctions) when it is in fact the reverse.

   Thus in planning a letter about a clinical session, it helps to be as clear as possible in one's thinking about *how much* of the work is being directed by the clinician and *how much* of it is consultative, i.e. based on consulting the client, about what has been decided and what remains to be considered. The point is that the letter, even in modest ways (e.g. drawing attention to a disagreement) should reflect – report and record – both sides of this balance.

2 Keep the letter consultative. A letter should not be directive, prescriptive or break new ground unless part of its purpose is to reflect this aspect of a session. Even then, its style and wording should convey such consultation as went on as well, which is largely about generating questions, curiosity and options. For example, consultation about whether to proceed with one therapy or another might lead to the patient asking the therapist to make the decision. This is a perfectly reasonable outcome of consultation – not the decision itself, but negotiated agreement about who is to decide. ('Negotiations' can convey an impression of long drawn-out discussion; but I am referring to a particular therapeutic style, and unless a serious conflict or misunderstanding is discovered – which by definition deserves attention anyway – it should take only minutes, and can be reflected in the letter in a sentence or a phrase, for example, 'all things considered we agreed that I should write to the

Headmaster'.) If the session *was* prescriptive, then say so: for example, 'please continue the medication as I advised', etc.

The point of all this is not courtesy but clarity, on the assumption that letters should accurately reflect and support therapeutic work, that the work is likely to contain decisions led by the clinician and those led by the patient, and that how decisions are made is important not only ethically and legally but to sustain work efficiently (Steinberg, 1987, 1992a).

3   The letter is a link between sessions. It should therefore refer back to what was discussed in the last session. Its function as a link between sessions can also be affirmed by, for example, confirming pieces of work to be done in the next session. It may be appropriate (for example, if something is persistently ambiguous or otherwise too problematic to spell out) to suggest that the letter forms the agenda for the next visit. Or, a written reply can be invited, explicitly or by implication; for example, if matters are left in the air and another session hasn't been arranged.

If no further attendance is anticipated (for example, a letter to someone who has made it clear that further contact isn't wanted) the letter should be planned accordingly (see e.g. Letter 3, p. 28, and Letter 42, p. 108).

4   The envelope must be precisely addressed and marked 'Confidential', as should the letter itself. People move house; the address in the notes may be wrong; the landlord or an inquisitive neighbour might open the letter, and the way it is addressed should not provide any excuse for this; there can even be confusion about who the patient is, especially if other members of the family are being seen. Consequently, some thought should be given to whether or not to employ 'return' labels.

5   How to address the recipients personally (and whom to address) needs consideration. Similarly, how one signs off will vary with different letters.

6   Letters can teach. The expectation to teach, with its encouragement for self-help as well as understanding, should be central to the task of composing these letters.

7   Jargon. It would be nice to simply advise the avoidance of jargon. However, some technical language is routine and usefully concise, and in any case what seems like jargon to one person may be ordinary language to another. All one can do is to be alert to jargon, to use plain language where possible, and where a technical term is needed to attempt a short, plain English explanation of it.

8   The letter as a contract. The letter can confirm at least a provisional agreement about how to proceed, what needs to be done, and what further questions need to be asked, including encouraging the patient's and family's questions.

9   Keep it short. Not brusque – courtesies are important. Nor over-abbreviated, because some things do need a reasonably expanded explanation (for example, a scary or potentially misunderstood diagnosis or prognosis). But try to keep it to under a page.

10   Think of the typist. A notable aphorism which has been attributed to several different people (hence my reluctance to give credit where it might not be due) is: 'I'm sorry for writing such a long letter, but I didn't have time to write a short one.' Rambling into a dictaphone, diverting everything in pursuit of after-thoughts, being over-inclusive and repetitive may seem to get the chore underway more quickly than pausing first to think and plan the letter. The more constructive thought you have given the case – which is another way of saying the more you know what you are doing – the shorter and clearer your dictation or typing. This is well worth practising, as it has applications well beyond writing letters.

Here is another quotation I like and whose provenance I've lost, though it really applies to writing articles: *'Write, rewrite, rewrite, revise; make your paper as short as you can. Then make it still shorter.'*

Finally, but first, discuss with your typist how the work should best be presented for typing.

Letters

Benefits, risks and side-effects

Benefits

To summarise Chapter 1

1   The letter helps train thinking.
2   It helps train writing.
3   It provides a concise written guide to assessment and treatments.
4   The letter survives the session physically, and renders substantial and permanent feelings and relationships which were transitory. It is a solid symbol of something which might be helpful. It can capture and 'hold' something safely which is troubling, confusing, elusive or ambiguous until it can be dealt with. It contributes to continuity.
5   It is a record of a significant piece of work; it can be reread outside the session. It is a reminder.
6   More than a record, it can be a contract. In some cases, perhaps increasingly, it may be reread whether or not the writer wishes it. For this reason alone, it's worth gaining experience at getting it right.
7   It might make you more efficient at planning care; it can even be interesting.

Risks and side-effects

These are:

1   Litigation.
2   Problems with confidentiality.
3   Getting it wrong in black and white.
4   Loss of control of the circumstances – perhaps time, place, situation and mood – in which the letter's message is read.
5   Misunderstandings and unintended messages.

---

1   Some readers may prefer to go straight to the first letter, on page 24, and return to Chapter 2 later.

6   The letter as a substitute for the session instead of a supplement for therapeutic work, or dominating it.
7   The letter as a substitute for writing proper notes.
8   The letter as something to make the therapist feel better.

Litigation

A distinguished senior colleague (some years ago) was rather proud of 'never writing anything down' – he claimed to do as much of his work as he could in conversation, including by telephone, and thought this helped keep him out of trouble. I don't think this is good advice. The Medical Defence Union – among other good teachers – advises being straightforward, including about mistakes, and stresses the importance of making full, clear and contemporaneous notes. It does not advise against apologising where appropriate. On the other hand, a rush to what seems to be honesty could also result in an assumption of fault which may be not only premature but incorrect.

Traditionally, doctors have communicated with doctors without anxiety about disclosure, and the clinical focus was ordinarily fairly tightly medical. Now, however, many professions and disciplines need or claim an interest in what is going on, the clientele may be the family rather than the individual patient (e.g. in family therapy and childcare generally), and increasingly issues of general public concern arise: risk to a child or other family member, and competence and dangerousness generally.

In a letter, as in the rest of a patient's records, the therapist needs to maintain a balance between the following triad: what is accurate, for the record; what needs to be said to whom, for therapeutic purposes; and how to say it positively, clearly, courteously and confidentially within a delineated group, and without being defamatory.

Defamation is unjust damage to someone's reputation. In permanent form (e.g. in the notes, a dictaphone tape or a letter) it is known as *libel*. In transient form (e.g. conversation) it is called *slander*. A successful case for libel therefore involves a defamatory statement communicated to a third party (i.e. anyone other than writer and patient) and which is understood to refer to the patient, even if this is by implication rather than by name. Suggestions that the person concerned is incompetent at his or her job, immoral, dishonest or criminal are described by lawyers as particularly perilous. However, a comment honestly made and without improper motive and on a matter of potential public interest (i.e. something in which the public are entitled to be interested, whether or not they are) may be regarded as fair comment, that is, not libellous. An apparently innocent statement could be libellous by innuendo, however, for example mentioning a family's luxurious life-style while drawing attention to their having no obvious means of financial support. On the other hand, informing someone who needs to know (i.e. can help) if a child or indeed any other person is at risk is a requirement; such questions of course raise issues of confidentiality as well as libel, and offending against professional codes of confidentiality is probably a greater risk in day-to-day practice than libel.

To the extent that what is written reflects precisely the interchange in the session, which should also be guided by courtesy and ethics and common sense about the law, there ought not to be a problem. This is particularly so if – as I would advise – the letter isn't an 'extra' but is mentioned in the session, including its contents and to whom you would like to send copies. As is often the case, a clinical dilemma can be transformed into a manageable focus for work if it is given centre stage, rather than allowed to persist as a peripheral niggle (Steinberg, 1983, 1987). There is an example of this on page 51 *et seq.*

Incidentally, it is worth remembering that quite apart from any question of slander, criticism of a medical colleague is seriously frowned upon (in the United Kingdom) by the General Medical Council. A letter containing a second opinion, especially if also sent to a patient, may well include views differing from those of other practitioners, medical or otherwise, and a little care is needed here.

In the psychiatric, psychotherapeutic and psychosocial fields in particular, fact can blur with opinion, one man's orthodoxy can appear controversial to someone else, misunderstandings can occur, and the wrong things can be said, and neither our colleagues nor our clientele can be relied on to be invariably in a reasonable or generous frame of mind. Moreover, in medical work in general, and psychiatric care in particular, dilemmas, including reasonable ways of proceeding and questions of who needs to know what are increasingly complex and a source of dispute. The practitioner on the spot may have to make decisions about moral dilemmas and complex circumstances which a roomful of learned lawyers and experts would remain unsure about even after weeks of examination and enquiry.

These are deep waters. Fortunately, judges know this; they respect conscientious efforts to help that are made in difficult circumstances, and lawyers know that judges take this view. I think a practitioner whose letters reflect conscientiously conducted work has nothing to fear. However, it is nice not to have to go as far as the Courts for such reassurance and encouragement.

Meanwhile, keep up to date with the latest advice from professional bodies, including local advisory and audit groups. Black *et al.* (1998) provide a useful guide to legal and ethical aspects of child psychiatry, with special reference to writing formal reports to other agencies, and to the Courts, an important subject but one which isn't the focus of this book; see also Tufnell *et al.* (1996).

Problems with confidentiality

For doctors, the bald fact of confidentiality is that he or she can only talk about a patient's history and clinical state to another doctor, without first seeking permission. Even discussing a patient's case with the multidisciplinary team is not privileged; that is to say you cannot assume it is always alright, and that it could not be challenged on legal or ethical grounds. Against this there is (1) the right of 'needing to know', for example, a nursing team needing to know about a patient's treatment, and (2) situations where it is obvious, from the way discussion is going, that someone else is going to be involved, for example, an agreed referral, say, to a psychotherapist, social worker or educational psychologist. But ensure that this is obvious to the patient and family too. As I said earlier, the point of letters of the sort we are discussing here is to reflect the session, so difficulties over what may or may not be said should not be left until the patient and family have gone home and the writer is sitting alone in the clinic wondering what to put in the letter. *Consult the patient and family while they are there; any problem or dilemma is by definition a useful focus for work.*

Thus the best course is to involve the patient or family in discussing the broad themes you would like to put in the letter, and to whom you would like to send copies. If for any reason it isn't useful or feasible to think through your letter with your clientele, you will often find yourself entrusted to send the relevant information to appropriate third parties if you ask. But do ask. The time to seek written permission is when agreement is ambiguously given, and of course when writing to informants before the first appointment, when you do not yet know the people you are going to see, nor they you. However, whatever implied, explicit or assumed permission you have, your letters should be clearly marked 'Confidential'; and because whomever you write to, you cannot be sure *who* will open and read the letter, one should write in a way that, as far as possible, is not too much of a disaster if it falls into the wrong hands. If the reader perceives this as an impossible requirement, I can only agree, but I believe it helps establish trust to convey that one has thought about the matter, and to bear in mind that the object is therapeutic integrity, not 'covering oneself' absolutely and legalistically.

Common sense about confidentiality, fine tuned with vigilance and a preparedness to err on the side of caution, and with those helpful phrases *acting in good faith*, *acting in the best interests of the child* and *acting in the public interest* as guides, together make an occasionally difficult letter-writing task manageable.

I have already mentioned the importance of being quite sure where your letter goes to. A letter is likely to refer to matters that are very personal and extremely sensitive, however carefully you phrase it. Hence make sure it is properly addressed, and, if your patient lives in an environment where boundaries are blurred and there is little reliable privacy, you should be aware of this and take appropriate precautions. If a really difficult and private matter requires mention in a letter which could go astray, I would simply allude to 'the problem we discussed' and if possible give the person concerned the letter directly. Some patients, especially young ones, may need a reminder to look after it – far from being litigious or over-sensitive, many of our clientele are too trusting and open, if not careless. 'Return labels' can be helpful in enabling the Post Office to send undelivered letters back to you, and with a little imagination a small sticky label can be produced that doesn't give away your specialty, which is a private matter between you and your client.

Getting it wrong in black and white

This very obvious risk is worth acknowledging. If you refer to Darryl's mother as Mrs Brown when she is actually Tania Baker, Jim's partner; or if you thought someone had been helped by a prescription which had nearly killed him, such misunderstandings may be swiftly put right in conversation, but will look clumsy in the extreme in writing. Family circumstances in child and adolescent psychiatry can be particularly complex, with Uncle Reggie not really being related to the patient, the partner who accompanies a parent and child not being the partner who is ordinarily at home, and several siblings having different surnames from each other and from the parents. It is a courtesy as well as essential for proper care to get such things right. People know when their lives are unusually complicated, and if for any reason (especially if you aren't a family therapist or social worker) you aren't sure precisely whom you saw and who was waiting outside in the car, phone or write and say so (with a stamped return envelope), explaining that you want to get relationships (or whatever) right in order to write to them properly. This will not seem ridiculous but sensible.

Loss of control of the circumstances

Most people in the therapeutic and caring professions dislike this. The fact is that one way or another, whether obviously or with apparent insouciance, we like to keep a firm grip on the situation when we see our clientele, and to make fine adjustments as we go along, including correcting misunderstandings. A comment, interpretation or piece of information is likely to be given in a carefully timed way; this is a crucial clinical skill. The letter, however, may arrive, or be read, or reread, or read 'properly', at any time, including in moods and circumstances that the writer might regret. This is why the letter itself should be finely judged, written for as wide a range of circumstances as possible – particularly moods – and reasonably formal. Do not attempt wit unless you are quite sure how it will be received.

Misunderstandings and unintended messages

This is not quite the same point as the one above. Leaving aside the risk of the atmosphere in which the letter is read not being the one you were writing for, a misperception which can be handled positively in the consulting room (for example, dealing skilfully with an angry, paranoid or fear-laden reaction) has no such chance of being put right when the patient is alone with the letter. Anyone can read between the lines correctly or otherwise, or read something into a phrase or sentence which wasn't intended. Nor does it have to be a major matter. A very obvious mistake is likely to be pointed out, but even if the finer points of a problem are given the wrong emphasis this can undermine confidence and the therapeutic relationship.

The letter as a substitute for the session

The letter should supplement therapeutic work, and not deal with new matters which should have been the focus of work in the session. The exceptions are when the writer judges that it will be helpful to use a narrative technique, opening up further something already identified with the patient and exploring it in writing, or when he or she thinks that an issue in the session should have been given more emphasis (or becomes aware of a mistake) and wants to mention it as something to be thought about between sessions and discussed next time. It's best not to get into the position where there is a need to write about a completely new topic or something important which one forgot to mention, such as the side-effect of a drug, or that someone else will be taking your clinic next time; however, such things happen, and, with a little thought, something therapeutic can be made of it.

Having said all this, it is of course reasonable to use letters as substitutes for sessions when the patient will not attend but needs some contact. Examples are given later.

The letter as a substitute for writing proper notes

This is a tricky one. Longhand notes can not only be tiresome, but unrewarding for their future readers. It is tempting to cram as much as possible into a dictated letter to save scratching away with a pen for half an hour or more. Some consultants begin a three- or four-page letter along the lines that 'you already know the history, but, for the sake of the record . . . '. I have done this myself; it can be appropriate, especially for complex, long-standing cases where the particular way in which the writer perceives the clinical story as developing and unfolding seems worth setting down.

There are also letters, not particularly from doctors, I would add, that give every twist and turn of several sessions' conversation in a five- or six-page letter. They are sometimes handwritten, and make no real attempt at a summary; there is sometimes evidence in the document that it is doing service as an all-purpose, multiple-recipient letter as well as being something for the record. (On the other hand, some letters are so taciturn that one is left feeling one is intruding in some way by wanting to know more). All one can advise, rather optimistically, is to write proper case records and proper letters.

The letter as something to make the therapist feel better

Therapy of any sort is a complex transaction. Being human, therapists do what they do partly for themselves and partly for others, and often enough the patient benefits too. All clinical and therapeutic training which has learned anything from psychodynamic thinking allows for those aspects of the work which are essentially for the sanity, safety and self-esteem of the therapist. This includes feelings of countertransference (the feelings the patient provokes in the therapist, and which can usefully guide therapy), activity that has to do with administration and organisation (including its academic aspects), legal and ethical considerations, and maintenance strategies that are primarily used to sustain and contain the work and keep it on course. 'Fallout' from any of this can find its way into letters.

An example of the sort already mentioned is to bring up or stress something in a letter which was neither mentioned nor emphasised in the session, possibly because it was difficult for some reason. For example, the therapist might have double-booked a session, be planning a holiday at the 'wrong' time, leaving, or a change involving another key member of the team may be about to happen. Or the therapist may think that a patient needed more advice than was given in the session about a specific risk – for example, from their own behaviour, from a relative or from newly prescribed medication. A serious omission in one of the above categories may well require correction and a brief explanation (and apology, if appropriate) about why it has been raised in a letter.

However, there are more subtle infelicities in therapy which should be corrected in a further session rather than by letter: for example, it would be wrong to write a strongly worded letter about an adolescent's (or anyone else's) misbehaviour if, in the session, the therapist let it pass with a mild admonition or none at all. If it *really* needs mentioning in a letter, it is probably best to identify it as something forgotten or omitted for some other reason, rather than letting it seem to be no more than a casual afterthought. It should also be mentioned as something to be discussed in the next session.

The letters in *Chapter 3* are about writing to patients and others at the very beginning of work, and concern not only first impressions of the therapist or service but give some indication of how clientele are handled and responded to. It includes examples of writing to non-attenders, including people who hadn't expected to be involved.

The letters in *Chapter 4* represent letters to the referring clinician but with a copy to the patient and family, yet written as much for the latter as for the doctor. I or my secretary first checks that the doctor concerned is happy about this, and in any case I send the briefest of covering notes; but essentially, one letter provides the information for all concerned.

Chapters 5 and 6 represent general maintenance: getting the work to the right altitude and keeping it there. There are examples of attempts to correct a first appointment that misfired, or work that suddenly took a downward turn; keeping the work on track when events (sometimes dramatic improvements) threaten to abort it; suggesting a change of course or an end to treatment; keeping communication open in uncertain situations; maintaining continuity between sessions (including suggestions about bringing up something new), and reviewing progress and aims.

Chapter 7 is about selected special situations: a complaint; a second opinion conveying a major change of direction; responding to a request to leave the family doctor out of the picture; trying to help an ex-patient persevere with someone else's care; the diagnosis to include on an insurance form; and, just to illustrate that *nothing* need be taboo in psychiatric and psychotherapeutic circles in 2000, asking about an unpaid bill.

Chapter 8 is about endings, and includes responding to a letter of thanks and letters about further or alternative care.

Outlining the letters thus does rather make them resemble a collection of 'how to say it' letters. I appreciate the risk of their coming across this way, but that isn't really the point of this book. Rather, I have tried to cover a range of some forty or so situations (and their multiple sub-themes) as a focus for a far wider task that is pivotal in our work: finding the right word.

Chapter 3

Beginnings

Invitations to the clinic

1 Changing times

Dear Mr and Mrs Baker, Clare and James,[1]

Thank you for your message, Mrs Baker,[2,3] to my secretary. I can change our next appointment from 2.30 to 3.30 p.m. on Friday 23rd next, and look forward to seeing you then.

Yours sincerely,

Derek Steinberg[4]
Consultant in Child and Adolescent Psychiatry[4]

Notes

1 Mr and Mrs Baker have made it clear that they would like to be known to me as Terry and Maggie, which is what Clare, who is 16, and James, 11, call them. I believe that what we call each other has an impact on our professional relationship and therefore on the treatment, and deserves a little thought.
2 It was Mrs Baker who relayed the message about the change of appointment for our first session after the initial assessment. There had been some difficulty about confirming the time of this second session, with Mr or Mrs Baker twice calling on their own or on another family member's behalf to explain that they couldn't after all make the appointment agreed to. I have responded to this slight but recurring turbulence by writing back each time to confirm the latest appointment, and addressing the whole family regardless of who called.
3 On the other hand, it can be quite useful, if slightly clumsy, to address one member of the family within a letter addressed to all. This is appropriate here, as it was Mrs Baker who phoned.
4 How to sign off is as important as how to address people, and I ring the changes from time to time, with the above as the standard. However, it seemed to me that if my name and job title recurred throughout the book this would be repetitive to the point of becoming tiresome. Most of the letters therefore end as I end them when

dictating to my secretary, with 'Yours sincerely, etc.'. Variations are printed more fully, with the reasons. In this case I signed off with my first name too, as I usually do.

Comments

I call adolescent patients by their first names, and their parents and adult patients usually Mr, Mrs or whatever. For the general purposes of this book I will simply acknowledge that all clinicians and other therapists have their own feelings and rules about this, and many simply go by what feels right at different times and with different people.

In Clare's case (she being the identified patient) it felt wrong to accede to her parents' request. It had something to do with the jolly heartiness of the first session; indeed, it began in the waiting room and continued along the corridor. The referring doctor had said in his first referral letter what a delightful family they were, and that he was at a loss to understand Clare's depression. He too used everyone's first names, as it turned out that he and the family were good friends. The beginning of the first session was marked by our all beaming delightedly at each other, not something that was easy to opt out of, because, as the family doctor had said, they were indeed nice people.

Now, one of the frustrations for the reader more than the writer of this book is that it will only be realistic to outline the case histories, and in many examples I will simply extract a fragment of a patient's case to explain the thinking behind something in a letter. Providing the full story would not only have doubled the size of the book but would distract from its focus, which is the letter and not the case history.

In Clare's case, as some may have suspected, role-blurring and problems with parental authority – indeed adulthood – turned out to be a key problem. As an adolescent, Clare was dealing with being different from her parents; her parents, however, for reasons which later emerged from their own backgrounds, wanted to thoroughly enjoy Clare's adolescence along with her, as participants. They were hurt and saddened whenever Clare tried to distance them from teenage parties and trips, despite their generous help in their organisation, funding, assistance and so on. Clare, when referred, was sad, angry and, above all, confused, not least because in whichever direction she tried to be an individual this challenged the image of the perfect family. As the origins of her distress emerged (to the parents' hurt astonishment), she talked in terms of feeling robbed. There were other important and difficult matters too, including the expectation that Clare would be the perfect scholar ('but she knows we only want for her what she wants for herself'), and James having a similar role in the family but one which, at age 11, he was still rather enjoying. He was *appreciative*, unlike Clare.

Without making too much of it, I believe that adopting 'Dear Mr and Mrs' and declining 'Terry and Maggie' helped set the tone for the difficult work of re-establishing parental authority and Clare's experiments with autonomy; and that the opposite would have set us all off at the wrong angle.

2 An invitation to the clinic

Dear Mr and Mrs Johnson, Alan, Barbara and Martin,[1, 2]

As you know we have been asked to see Alan and would like to offer an appointment at 2 p.m. on Thursday 18 March here at this clinic. We would like to meet everyone who is living together at home. Please be prepared to spend about an hour and a half with us, as its important that we make adequate time to deal with all your concerns.[3, 4]

We operate as a multidisciplinary team[5] and during the afternoon you may meet one of our social workers as well as a clinical psychologist, occupational therapist, one of the teachers from our school and one of the nursing team from our residential unit, as well as the consultant in child and adolescent psychiatry. We are part of a teaching hospital, and there may be one or two people present who are training in one of the above professions. Some of them will observe our interviews from behind a screen, but you will meet them first and have the opportunity to express any concerns about this that you may have. The interviews will also be recorded with your permission.[6]

We find it helpful if we can contact anyone who has previously seen Alan, and would be grateful if you would return the enclosed form listing them, please signing your permission for us to get in touch. As Alan is 16 he will need to sign too.

We have allotted Nikki to be your key worker, please don't hesitate to contact her with any queries or concerns.[3, 4, 7]

We look forward to meeting you and doing our best to help.

Yours sincerely,

Nikki Smith   Jim Brown   Mike Watson
Psychologist   Senior Social Worker   Consultant Psychiatrist

Notes

1   This sort of letter used to be duplicated, with gaps left so that the patient's name and other details could be filled in. In some ways this format had more integrity, being very obviously impersonal, duplicated for convenience, and somewhat ramshackle. The word processer, however, provides a seamless pretence of being a personal letter, a mild deception which everyone recognises, especially when jarred by its infelicities.

2   What do Barbara and Martin know about Alan's problem, the referral and the clinic, for example? Will they see the letter? It also happens that Martin is 4 months old; the referral letter simply mentioned that Alan had an older sister and a younger brother. A cousin, Susan, aged 13, a troubled girl, is currently staying with them for

an indefinite period, because of a crisis in the extended family. As the letter says, Nikki, Jim and Mike would like to see everyone. However, different services have different policies about how many members of the family they expect to see, or even insist on seeing, particularly at the first session. The catch-all style of the letter doesn't properly deal with this. Who is addressed in this first letter, and how – as clearly the family is quite unknown to Nikki, Jim and Mike – needs more thought and preparation than this letter demonstrates.

3   The importance of making 'adequate time to deal with all your concerns' conveys that nice mixture of earnest helpfulness, bossiness and slight menace that can characterise our helping and caring professions. 'Concerns' is very PC (see p. 9), all other words (e.g. worries, anxieties, problems, difficulties) tending to be considered as rather presumptive and undemocratic if not frankly authoritarian, while 'concerns' is egalitarian and neutral to the point of disappearing.

4   The misspelt 'its' and the rather breathlessly clumsy '. . . key worker, please don't hesitate' (there should be a full stop or a semicolon.) is shoddy. Therapists and clinicians should be thoughtful, careful and precise, particularly about words, and our literature should demonstrate this. On this point, the quality and design of the clinic stationery should be good. This need not be expensive.

5   Much of this paragraph sounds like a mission statement hammered out by the team, and this phrase is a good example. It has something of a charter or contract about it, one that may be designed as much to keep team members in their place as the clientele. The referrer possibly explained to Alan or his parents that he was going to see a social worker, a psychologist, a doctor or 'experts who help young people with this sort of thing', but usually the team don't know how the referrer has described the service. Hence this all-purpose self-description, which may satisfy a need within the team but doesn't really explain or inform, beyond giving an impression of a busy and perhaps rather organisationally important routine.

6   Is this an instruction, a request or a warning?

7   The informality of the use of first names contrasts with the highly controlling tone of the letter.

Comments

This is a very poor letter, but many clinics use something similar. I have been involved in producing this sort of document myself, and I've no doubt shared responsibility from time to time for something very much along these lines.

Working with children and adolescents is complex, and what it involves in general and how it will work in practice for the referred patient and family isn't that easy to convey concisely in the best of circumstances. I think it is valuable for a specialised service to prepare:

1   a standard and thoughtfully written printed leaflet briefly describing the specialty in general and the way this particular service works, and explaining how work with new clientele gets under way. It can list staff members, and probably provide a simple map with bus routes and so on.

2   If needed, a simple written statement about confidentiality and ethics may accompany a form for the patient and parents to return, and which could provide space for questions as well as for giving permission to liaise with others.

3   A short, friendly, personal letter, preferably from one person (for example, the staff member whom they will meet on the day and who will take a lead in the first interview), confirming the appointment and approximately how long it is likely to take, and mentioning any enclosed leaflets that describe the service.

A letter like this could mention one or two other people who are expected to be there, but my own feeling about letters signed by several people is that there is something creepily cautious about them, as if they aren't quite used to trusting each other. I wouldn't like to receive a similar letter from a surgeon and his team, though some might.

3 A reluctant attender

Dear Michael,[1]

As you know, your parents came to see me the other day to discuss their worries about you. I'm sorry you decided not to see me yourself. I know your parents tried hard to persuade you, and that this caused yet another big argument, but I think they were right to try, even though you are old enough to make the final decision yourself.[2]

This does leave me with a problem, though.[3] Your parents are worried about how things are at home and they want to see me. I do think I should see them at least a few times to see if there is any way of my helping them[4] put right some of the things they think they are getting wrong.[5] I think they are entitled to my advice if they want it, although I appreciate it must feel like you are being discussed behind your back.[6]

I will therefore go ahead with offering to see your parents on this basis.[7]

If you decide, some time, that you would like to come along for one of the meetings, please check with them first, because these next few appointments are primarily for them.[8] If you do come, I think it will help.

If you would prefer a word with me first, just ring my secretary and let me know.[9]

Yours sincerely, etc.[10, 11]

Notes

1 Michael is aged 17 and has every right not to see me, indeed not to have anything to do with the clinic. I glimpsed him when he came as far as the waiting room, protesting, on the first occasion, before going off to wait for his parents outside. I addressed this letter to him, and not to Michael and his parents, although a different sort of letter could have addressed all three. I marked it 'Confidential'.

2   This first paragraph acknowledges Michael's rights, but his parents' rights too.

3   I too have my rights and my problems in this situation, and I thought it would help to remind Michael, who I judged to be fearful as well as angry, that my own position has its dilemmas too, one of which is that I want to find a way to help.

4   This statement is guided by ethics and actuality, not compromise. To try to 'manage' Michael by proxy would be improper, I think, as well as clinically risky. My letter and chosen way of proceeding assumes that he is essentially a reasonable young man, albeit anxious, angry and unhappy, and my remit is to try to help two parents manage the situation at home under these circumstances.

5   This statement affirms both that I will be working with the parents' difficulties, not his, and that they believe, with help, they could handle things better; it isn't all for Michael to put right.

6   As well as refusing to come along, Michael is also putting pressure on his parents not to talk about him behind his back. While (5) addresses this, it seemed right to acknowledge the issue in this way too, and, without risking mockery or accusation, to use his own words. (Thus it would have been a mistake, I think, to have quoted him between inverted commas.)

7   Having talked around the matter, it then seemed right to make a clear statement of my decision.

8   This reminds Michael that he is also someone who can make decisions, and also that the situation has now changed. I will be seeing his parents; the appointments are not now for him. But the situation can revert to what I think is the preferable one.

9   I don't yet have a relationship with Michael, and don't yet know quite what his relationships are with his parents. I therefore wanted him to have two routes back to the clinic from which to choose. I also felt that the phrase 'have a word' conveyed the possibility of an adult conversation, if he felt he could use it.

10 This is a note about something not in the letter. This young man, old enough to refuse treatment (unless desperately ill) and with an unknown mental state, could have been reminded about the availability of his own GP if he didn't want to talk to me or his parents. It would have covered all eventualities, at least in a letter, but it would have felt more like something to reassure me (p. 21) than help Michael. Suggesting a third option would seem, I thought, to risk devaluing the main suggestions: to talk to his parents or to talk to me.

11 It crossed my mind to write a shorter letter, though not a longer one. As it stands it is somewhat repetitive. However, I didn't think its length would have materially affected whether or not it went straight into the waste bin.

Comments

This situation is not uncommon in adolescent psychiatry, but it has its adult versions too, and these can be even more alarming. At one extreme it may turn out that a reluctant clinician sees a reluctant patient who has nothing wrong with him or her apart from over-anxious or intrusive relatives. At the other extreme the clinician may be told about someone unwilling to come along who might (but might not) be on the point of committing suicide or homicide. This typically presents on a Friday evening, when most of the rest of the world seems to have gone home. The issue is not how to predict the future on the basis of inadequate information, but of weighing one set of risks against the other. (In other words, to *really* raise anxiety, to act in a way which you would not be embarrassed about describing to your lawyer.) One of my observations in this situation was that Michael had come along with his parents despite the rows that had preceded the appointment, had waited in the waiting room until I asked to see them, and waited outside until they took him home again. There was a sustainable relationship there, albeit a currently turbulent one, which told me something about Michael as well as about his parents. When I saw them, I asked them some clinical questions which led me to suspect that Michael was depressed and angry but not desperate, and that a likely component of the problem lay in family relationships. It didn't appear to me to be likely that Michael had a psychotic illness – at least not an obvious one – or that he had a profound personality disorder, or was physically ill. On balance, therefore, it seemed reasonable to proceed through working with his parents while trying to engage Michael by letter.

Another letter I had to write was to the referring family doctor to let her know I was seeing not Michael but his parents. I sent her a copy of my letter to Michael, which I thought was the best way of putting her in the picture about the management plan that was emerging.

The next session involved my exploring a number of fairly common-sense strategies about how Michael's parents could respond to his increasing rebellious-ness; he had a part-time job and was on a part-time vocational course, doing both moderately well, and leaving home hadn't occurred to anyone as an option. However, he was raising hell there, bringing home alcohol, drinking heavily and going around with a marginally delinquent group, all this representing a relatively sudden change in his character and life-style of two years before. His father had become unemployed about two years before that, and subsequently quite depressed, which he still was, and which showed itself, among other ways, in his lack of optimism about any strategy we (he, his wife and I) might develop for managing Michael, which was based in turn on his own lack of confidence about sustaining anything which was even slightly challenging. His wife responded by unwillingly, angrily and ineffectively taking the lead. The focus shifted from what to do for Michael to what to do for his father, and, when Michael began to join in the sessions (he came to the third one and took a full part, in some respects acting as the man of the family), he made it increasingly clear that he thought his parents needed help before he did. He was intrigued by the notion that he might have engineered things this way by misbehaving and then refusing to accept outside help.

The letter had been intended to be no more than stating a way of proceeding in an uncertain situation, while hoping that Michael would either come along or not feel the need to. However, by affirming a common-sense plan (more consultative than clinical) of exploring what was feasible, it wasn't inconsistent with what some-what unexpectedly followed: the emergence of Michael's strengths, his father's difficulties and his mother's predicament, quite helpfully as it subsequently turned out.

4 Extra help needed

Dear Mrs Wright,

I think you know that your daughter Joanna and her three children have been referred to me by their family doctor.[1] We have now seen them three times, that is myself and the community psychiatric nurse who works with me, and although things have been very difficult we have now started to make some real progress.[2] Unfortunately Joanna and the children, especially Jamie, are bothered by divided loyalties. They didn't want to tell me what the problem was about, in fact they seemed quite embarrassed, but my impression is that you thought it was unnecessary for your daughter to seek advice about Jamie's behaviour, and that you've been quite upset by the fact that they are now attending a child psychiatric clinic.[3] It seems that when I suggested that Joanna ask you to come along for us all to discuss things together, this led to a very upsetting argument, and I'm sorry if my suggestion was the cause of that. However, I'm worried about Joanna feeling pulled in two directions, and quite apart from her own feelings about this the children do definitely need consistent handling. Joanna wants and needs your help and support, but it does seem she wants ours too.[4] I would also be interested to hear your point of view too, about how things have got difficult between Joanna and the children, and the best way of helping. I would be grateful if you could find time to come along to one of the sessions to talk over some of these issues, and of course for my colleague here and I to answer any questions you have about what we do.

I should say that Joanna didn't really want me to write this letter, thinking it would upset you, though she does agree that we can't leave things just as they are.[4] However, I did persuade her to let me send it, as long as you were the only person who saw it.[5] If you agree to meet us, please just come along with Joanna. If you prefer, give me a ring whether you want to come along or not.

With best wishes.

Yours sincerely, etc.[6]

Notes

1 We could have plunged straight in with the second sentence, affirming what we and the family were engaged in. This tentative beginning felt right however; it acknowledged that Mrs Wright was at some distance from the situation and yet did have some involvement in it. It was an attempt, probably unconscious as far as the choice of words went, to give her *distancing* of herself something of the flavour of *standing back* instead. Monitoring her antagonism here would have been superfluous.

2 It was proper to inform her as a sceptical person that there had been progress with big problems; Joanna, the nurse and I were getting somewhere, hence had some authority in this matter and deserved a hearing.

3 Although this is put politely enough, i.e. that Mrs Wright's views might be as good as ours, it wasn't really what we suspected, which was that she was undermining

Joanna and messing up our management plans. In fact the more positively framed part of the phrasing turned out to be nearer the truth, and her contribution to be real, and valuable. Thus the rather ambiguous framing of the matter for discussion – 'thought it was unnecessary' – really did enable Mrs Wright's contribution.

4 We were in difficulties over Joanna's mixed feelings. She was very young – 20 – and wanted to manage by herself, yet wanted help too; she perceived Mrs Wright partly as a helpful parent and partly as an ogre. Joanna's father had left home during her early teens. At this stage we didn't know who would end up being more influential in Joanna's life – ourselves or Mrs Wright. Ethically and legally, we could only send this letter with her informed consent, and we were satisfied, in the event, that we had it. On grounds of privacy and humanity we wanted her whole-hearted consent, and we were sure we had that too. But persuasion (to negotiate about it and listen to our explanations) had played its part, and we thought it right to mention this. It was true, but it also avoided causing a rift between Joanna and Mrs Wright should our own intervention go pearshaped.

5 Privacy was more the issue than confidentiality: see comments, below.

6 I had a co-worker. Notwithstanding the discussion on page 28, a joint signature is exactly right for many sorts of joint work. But we decided that I would write the letter in the first person, as psychiatrist, to tackle Mrs Wright's avowed antipathy to psychiatry head-on.

Comments

This case was quite a mess, and it took some time to sort out who was related to whom, despite the help of several social workers who had been involved over the years. The problem was that by the time we had tidied it up, so to speak, to try to focus help where it was needed, i.e. to support Joanna in her self-esteem and handling of her three quite difficult little boys, we had managed to exclude Mrs Wright from the situation, and she was angered by this.

The children had three different fathers, all now completely out of the picture. However, all three had relatives and children by other women and Joanna was in a complex, chaotic network of some twenty or more people and children who, as she saw it, helped or hindered her in their various ways.

Jamie's father, who had been particularly violent towards Joanna and the other children was now serving quite a long prison sentence. Mrs Wright lived on the other side of the district. She was a strong, kindly but overprotective woman, felt guilty about her problematic relationship with Joanna and the children, and visited Joanna's flat quite often, though not always welcome, doing her best to help out. Joanna had very mixed feelings about her, and at first didn't want her involvement until she saw that we would help her control it.

Mrs Wright was bitter about one of her nephews' experience of the psychiatric services. He sounded a very disturbed young man, though it seemed he hadn't attracted any particular diagnosis. He was eventually convicted of a serious assault while drunk and on drugs. His mother, Mrs Wright's younger sister, had taken him, or he'd been sent, to a number of psychiatrists, psychologists and others throughout his childhood and adolescence, and her perception was that they had all been unhelpful, rather as she had expected. Mrs Wright had been very close to her sister, who had responded to her efforts to intervene and help by blaming her for the outcome. She thought her nephew had been ill in some way, though in due course she had become completely disillusioned with 'psychiatry' (with which she lumped together other children's services). She was horrified when Joanna embarked on this route, particularly since it was Mrs Wright in the first place who had urged Joanna to take Jamie to the doctor because of stomach pains.

We didn't know these background details until we met Mrs Wright, which perhaps was just as well. The letter I sent made her feel, as she told me, that its writer had seemed 'fairly sensible', which is why she agreed to come along. There was a lot of anger and sadness to deal with, and family reconstituting to do, which included helping Joanna and Mrs Wright to deal with their respective losses, and to maintain a helpful distance between them. Once we had Mrs Wright 'on board', some quite straightforward behavioural strategies were put in place to help the children, following which Joanna was freed up to use a series of individual sessions with the community psychiatric nurse, and this helped a great deal.

All this, as they say, wasn't the half of it. However, it seemed that our rather simplistic letter, dropped into a complex and chaotic case which we were struggling with in a somewhat ramshackle way, served as a catalyst to tidy things up and render them potentially manageable; or rather, it had enabled Mrs Wright to become the somewhat unexpected catalyst and she moved from feeling shame about what had happened to her family (hence our emphasis on privacy helped) to be pleased at having helped put things right.

Chapter 4

Writing for referrer and patient

5 Twenty-second opinion

Dear Dr Singh,

Re: Robert ——— , aged 20, and address,

Thank you for asking me to see Robert.

I agree that Robert shows some features of autistic spectrum disorder of the relatively milder sort, and that he has some learning problems too along the lines described in the recent psychological assessment. Some of the experiences he reports complicate the clinical picture, but in my opinion they don't amount to psychotic symptoms. Rather, they reflect a preoccupation with science fiction imagery and ideas, not uncommon in his age group, but which he reports and perhaps experiences too in a somewhat literal way, because of his problems in self-expression. He is also somewhat obsessive, and his rather incontinent repetition of these ideas, sometimes at socially inappropriate times, causes alarm. However, I am quite satisfied that Robert regards them as his own ideas, i.e. he doesn't attribute them as coming from elsewhere, and my interpretation of the fact that he doesn't welcome all of them is simply that he has adolescent fantasies that are obsessive and which embarrass and upset him. These and other thoughts sometimes bring him to a halt, while he ruminates about them and tries to deal with them by repetitive rituals, and at such times he looks withdrawn, preoccupied and odd, and gets angry and incoherent if the rituals are interrupted. All this is consistent with obsessional thinking in a young man with limited self-expression, empathy and social skills, rather than with a schizophrenic illness.

I agree that there is really nothing that should be done for Robert which isn't being done already, and by an experienced team too, though I am not surprised that his progress, though real, is slow. One can understand his parents being anxious to leave no stone unturned, especially for a young man of only 20. The trouble is that his parents do not feel reassured that everything physical as well as psychological has ever been sufficiently investigated, or that there isn't another sort of approach or a new treatment that will make all the difference. He has had all the appropriate investigations and assessments for all of these, plus just about every treatment it is reasonable to try. However, their anxieties about Robert go back a long way, as you know, and I suspect that the recurring breakdown they have in their relationships with professionals is because their sense of bitterness and loss and their fears for the future have never been entirely taken up. I think it is important that someone tries, although it can be difficult to pursue this when they are thinking more in terms of medical diagnoses and solutions. As Dr Miles said in her report, the few drugs that seemed to help him a little also made him drowsy, but it does seem that the most help was with the milder tranquillisers at low dosage, which confirms my impression that anxiety rather than a psychotic condition is one of his key problems.

I think it would be best for Robert and his parents to stay with Dr Miles and her team, and for him to remain a termly boarder at S—— College for as long as they will have him, despite their feeling they aren't quite set up for his needs. I have told Robert and his parents that I don't advise any tests or new drugs, and there is indeed nothing I could advise specifically for Robert that hasn't been tried adequately already, but that I did think it would help if they talked over their disappointment with the social worker on Dr Miles' team. I have to say that they didn't think much of this suggestion, but thanked me for my time. I would be surprised if they don't come back to you again about seeing Dr K, whose clinic has had some more publicity recently. I'm sorry that there's nothing more I can suggest.

With best wishes.

Yours sincerely, etc.

Note

Although this is a fairly mediocre letter, and a bit too long, it would do. However, I think a better approach to helping Robert and his parents would be as follows:

Dear Dr Singh,

Thank you for asking me to see Robert. I would like to send a copy of the enclosed rather lengthy[1] letter to Robert and his parents. Could you kindly let my secretary know if you would be happy about this?

Best wishes.

Yours sincerely, etc.

Enc.

Dear Dr Singh,

Thank you for asking me to see Robert and his parents, and for sending me the helpful summaries from Dr Miles and from the others who have seen Robert. I spent some time with Robert, and then had a longer meeting with his parents, after which I saw them together. The enclosed letter contains the essence of what we discussed, and with your agreement I have sent them a copy.

Yours sincerely, etc.

c.c. Dr Miles

Dear Dr Singh,[2]

Re: Robert ——

Thank you for asking me to see Robert, whom I saw, separately and together with his parents, this morning. Thank you also for the set of very full summaries which you have passed on from Dr Miles.

Our discussion focused on two main issues. First, whether or not Robert has schizophrenia, a term which he and his parents were familiar with and worried about. Second, whether everything possible was being done for his condition.

I went through the story of Robert's development and the history of his problems from the family and from the notes, and spent some time with Robert by himself. The impression I had was of a pleasant, forthright young man, very able in some things (e.g. when doing practical things with clear instructions) but tending to get muddled and anxious in others (e.g. on social occasions or when he is expected to make decisions). For example, he enjoys gardening, keeps careful records, and does it well, but feels awkward and quite tense when with other young people at his college or when he meets young relatives and the children of his parents' friends. He has been so upset on some of these occasions in the past year that he has begun to avoid them.

As you know, some problems in Robert's early development are thought to have dated from some difficulties in his mother's pregnancy, something that has been mentioned several times in the family but I think not fully discussed, at least not in a way Robert can recall. He then had some problems with speaking and reading and with making friends and going to school, and two things started about then which have continued on and off ever since. First, Robert's tendency to double-check things in his head, which can last for some minutes, at which times he looks withdrawn, which of course he is, although he gets very frustrated and angry if people try to interrupt him. Second, and Robert says this is connected to what he checks in his head, he feels he has to tell people about some of the very odd ideas that occur to him, many of them connected with science fiction characters, aliens and so on. He is quite clear that these ideas, including what the characters say, and other noises (like flying saucers taking off) are made up by himself, even though he finds some of the ideas scary and they worry him at night. My impression was that Robert is a shy young man, really quite imaginative in some ways but not knowing what to do with or how to enjoy the ideas that occur to him, and quite troubled by this and by his difficulties in relationships with other young people.[4]

I have described Robert's problems in this way because, to me, they add up to a group of difficulties and disabilities rather than an illness. Robert knows about schizophrenia, and about autism and Asperger's syndrome, and about obsessive-compulsive disorder, and about learning problems, because, especially in recent years, the psychiatrists and psychologists he has seen and his parents have discussed these conditions with him. I think many of his problems most resemble Asperger's syndrome.

Different doctors have given different weights to these conditions in Robert's case over the years and, as far as I can tell, have applied all the appropriate treatments, but nothing has helped very much except the *lower* doses of those sedative drugs which didn't give him side-effects. Even they helped only a little.

What Robert and his parents are left with is a long list of possible diagnoses, but no treatment that has made a big difference to Robert, by which they mean his confidence, sense of happiness and his prospects of making friends and training for a reasonable job.[5] They quite correctly see Robert as handicapped in all these respects (though there has also been steady if slow progress over the years). They are quite worried about the possibility of a diagnosis being missed, especially a physical one (for example, one of the rare neurological disorders that have had a lot of publicity recently), or about new treatments from all the research that is going on not being tried.

I think they are absolutely right to wonder about such things, and to hope for a short cut to Robert making dramatic progress one day, but the chance of that – which, I have to say, I think is unfortunately small – has to be set against the risk of Robert and perhaps his parents as well feeling so frustrated with his slow progress that they don't always go along whole-heartedly with some of the approaches which I think *are* helping, for example, the family work,[6] the college's specialised educational programme (which quite impressed me), and the social skills training in small groups, which I know Robert finds difficult.

I don't think Robert has an active illness, by which I mean a mental or physical disorder like schizophrenia, that is acting on his mind and health day after day and which is still waiting for the right diagnosis and the right prescription. I think Robert did have something go wrong in his very early development, and it has left him with the sorts of problems in handling his thoughts, managing his feelings and coping with relationships that – with Robert's and his parents' help – I have outlined above.

I advised that the best way forward was, first, to concentrate on carefully focused training and education for all of Robert's difficulties, and this includes building on his very real strengths and abilities, rather than putting them on hold, so to speak, while waiting for the 'magic cure'.[7] I think the help he is getting from his college and from Dr Miles and her team is exactly right, and he is making steady progress. The one slight shift of emphasis I would suggest is to try treating Robert's problems in social settings more like a social phobia, for which there are techniques that Dr Miles' team would have available if they thought it could help.[8]

Second, Robert and his parents will benefit from reassurance that if anything unexpected came along, whether from Robert himself or from the researchers and other experts, its potential for helping Robert would of course be considered. Staying with the same team would be a good way of keeping everything under review.[9]

Third, all this needs trust, and trust needs to be worked at. Robert's parents have felt very let down over the years by the specialists they have seen, even though they say that for the most part they did their best. They just never seemed good enough or interested enough, to use their words, even though they couldn't put their finger on any particular complaint. If anything has needed more attention, in my opinion, it has been Robert's parents' feelings of anxiety, disappointment, failure and even grief; when Robert was very small they would worry all the time about whether he would survive; now they worry about whether he will ever be able to leave home, and as they say, they themselves aren't getting any younger; and another worry is that he is a big, strong, strapping chap[10] who might lose his temper in the wrong place or with the wrong people and get into serious trouble. Robert and his parents were glad that we broached these worries of theirs, but it wasn't easy at first, and they agreed that they couldn't easily imagine going into all these things for session after session. I said that I hoped the opportunity was still there, and that if they felt more comfortable seeing the social worker by themselves, without Robert, for some of the sessions, why not ask?

I thought there was a lot that could still be done for Robert, building on his strengths and on what is being done already by Dr Miles and the college,[11] although what I am suggesting isn't quite what Robert and his parents expected. They did agree with what I was advising, but frankly it isn't easy to raise all the questions one might like to at the end of a long session with a 'second opinion', and I took the liberty of suggesting that when the time felt right they should discuss this letter with Dr Miles or with yourself.[12]

Please let me know if you have any questions about it; I'm sorry it is so long.

With kind regards.

Yours sincerely, etc.

c.c.[3] Robert and Mr and Mrs ——
    Dr Miles

Notes

1 It is too long, and I have tried to make a number of points in one letter to illustrate the circumstances of more than one case. But there *are* cases with all these complexities, and, unfortunately, letters as long as this are kept in those tiny folders which general practitioners use. But there is a point to some of the circumlocutory phrasing and repetition. One is trying to help with a serious change in direction: from doubts, suspicions and bitterness about one specialist or team after another, always hoping there would be something they felt confident about around the corner, to dealing with anger, fears and doubts about doctors and nurses, themselves and Robert *from even before he was born*. Some careful explanation was therefore in order.

2 It occurred to me to address my letter to Robert and his parents; but I decided it would have more impact if it was addressed to Dr Singh and Dr Miles, so that whatever was being said between doctors was there for them to see, and I felt that there had to be this sort of impact for the change of direction that was needed. In addition, a letter addressed to the family would feel more like my being the next consultant in line than I would like. Having gone into Robert's case with them I believed my role should be to raise a question mark about seeking yet another specialist, and to encourage them to remain with their present sources of help. I wanted to stress that this was what I thought was right for Robert, in the light of seeing him, and them, and looking at the other teams' case notes. People do of course have an absolute right to second opinions, and often enough it is an unrecognised need; but when to stop? And how?

3 What about copying the letter to Robert himself, rather than to the family? He is old enough; but he came to see me with his parents, and it was they and the doctors who had initiated the second opinion. Had I been working with them, I think I would be making an early start on the independence issues that I have only alluded to in the letter. But I wasn't; as I said, I thought it was right to encourage them away from 'new' sources of help. Hence, if they reflected together over my letter, I assumed it would be as they were now, i.e. a close-family, and not as they might become in due course. On the other hand, it could be a good exercise to rewrite it from that perspective.

4 Expanding on how Robert came across in ordinary terms instead of clinical shorthand raises problems for the whole issue of writing such letters. Had I not been writing for Robert also, I think I would have described his mental state in textbook terms, noting, for example, the absence of delusions, hallucinations, thought insertion and passivity phenomena. Indeed, one might have conveyed the messages of the letter in about twenty lines. Although I was writing to Dr Singh and Dr Miles as if Robert and his parents were listening in, so to speak, it is really a letter to *them*, but for the reasons given above it was addressed to the doctors.

5 It seemed helpful to describe Robert's problems in plain language, as disabilities amenable to teaching and training, rather than as symptoms needing treatment. The former doesn't make it easier (in some ways it can be more difficult), but it renders the problems understandable, and potentially manageable by teachers and counsellors and other caregivers, unlike problems in brain chemistry which need psychopharmacologists and psychiatrists. But even when the latter is the case (e.g. in manic depressive illness and schizophrenia), there are always management and

self-management issues (like taking medication) that should be framed as centre-stage common-sense matters rather than as peripheral 'extras'.

6 In fact, Robert's parents have felt that attempts at family work have been substitutes for medical investigation and treatment, rather than part of compre-hensive clinical management, and moreover that they implied blame. I was quite sure that in addition, and at least as importantly, they had real and understandable difficulties about facing some long-term and very painful matters concerning themselves as individuals, as husband and wife and as parents. We went some way towards acknowledging this, enough, I thought, for the purposes of this consultation and letter. I wanted to frame the issue in words which were accurate enough, and which left the issue sufficiently open, but which would leave Robert's parents enough in control to take the risk of exploring their anger and grief.

7 'Magic cure' reflected well enough what Robert's parents had been hoping for, though as sensible, well-informed people they hadn't previously seen it in such terms. I used the phrase in the letter because it felt alright to do so following our discussion. But be very careful with quotes in quotation marks, which can come across as patronising or worse.

8 Apart from family therapy for disabling feelings of grief about failed reproduction, the other 'new' piece of advice is to treat some of Robert's anxiety and awkwardness as a social phobia. From what Dr Miles' team are doing, it is clear that they could adopt this suggestion if they wanted to, if, as I've put it, they thought it would help. The cautious phrasing and ambiguity – diplomacy if you like – is deliberate, and it reflects how I saw the situation, which is that while I did have something new to suggest, I also thought it vital that Dr Singh and Dr Miles should retain continuing medical authority.

9 There is more than one way to give advice; one doesn't have to be tentative and consultative. There are specific suggestions here about the importance of continuity for Robert's care, training and education, but the work of helping the family as a whole and Robert's parents in particular with their long-standing disappointment and frustration is going to take time even just to get started. There is also the suggestion to keep an eye open for something new, i.e. exactly what Robert's parents originally wanted – something undiscovered in his head, or a new treatment. However, my intention was to put it into an entirely different context: not as something to be sought while everything else is put on hold year after year, but as an important additional item in an elaborate management plan. There was also the reference to recognising the diagnosis of social phobia – about the only diagnosis Robert hadn't attracted thus far.

10 I have stressed real fears and real problems several times while attempting to place a more positive connotation alongside them. Thus describing Robert as a big, strapping chap (an avuncular, corny phrase; not one I liked, but it fitted) was a cosy counterbalance to his parents' fears that as he grows bigger and stronger and tries to be independent (with the help of the mixed sex social skills group at the college) they might live to see him in the newspapers as an arrested rapist or murderer. This frightening fantasy, not readily volunteered but acknowledged with considerable relief when it came up, surfaced every time there was some such report in the news.

11 Putting something in a positive light is also a reminder of those of Robert's qualities that are taken for granted as we all – Robert included – become

preoccupied with his problems. He is ninety per cent fine, if such things could be quantified, and his strengths need to be acknowledged to help him and his therapists and teachers to handle the ten per cent that isn't.

12 I was actually not sure whether either Dr Singh or Dr Miles would be the best person for Robert and his family to discuss the letter with; that's up to them. But I wanted to suggest that the letter contains things worth reflecting about with help, and that it might (in fact ought to) generate questions. If there are any questions for me, I would rather they came via one of the two doctors; again, to emphasise where I thought authority should remain: with Robert, his family and their present doctors; not with me.

Comments

Many of the points I want to make about Robert's case have been outlined in the above notes. This chapter is about letters intended to inform, and what I wanted to convey, as the 'second' opinion, was (1) something of a summary as I saw it of what had happened to date; (2) some definite suggestions about how to proceed, although deliberately framed to sustain the authority, responsibility and possibly the morale of those currently managing the situation, rather than suggesting that I should or even could take over myself; and (3) quite a big shift of emphasis, away from the hunt for a diagnosis and cure that will make all the difference, and towards what I thought was hampering Robert's progress: that his parents were stuck with an old issue, its origins in all sorts of hopes, fantasies, losses and disappointments to do with their lives from their teens to the time he was born twenty years ago. Appreciating and helping him as an individual was being hampered by a quietly frantic hunt for something that would put the clock back to before the frightening time when obstetricians and nurses started signalling that things might not be perfect, and paediatricians and later child psychiatrists tried to find encouraging words to say about Robert's increasingly obvious developmental troubles. The letter, I hoped, might at least lay the foundations for trying to help with these difficult and disabling long-term feelings.

Robert had been born after ten years' trying and two miscarriages, one of them quite late. For reasons which had their roots in Robert's parents' own lives, and indeed (as it emerged) in their choosing each other, success as man, woman, husband, wife and parents was emotionally very loaded. Robert as evidence of this was very important, and their worst anxieties were confirmed when Robert's development took them on a relentless trajectory further and further away from the ideal child and the ideal family. The established pattern became the wait in busy specialists' and social workers' waiting rooms, rather than enjoying school successes and exciting new friendships. The real difficulty for the professional workers of handling their shock and loss compounded matters. It couldn't be done by a friendly word alone, and the occasional time when someone happened to say just the right thing was spoiled by the many other well-meaning but rather clumsy things that were said. Either it needed something very old-fashioned, a real, close, sustained and understanding relationship with a friend or relative or a non-clinical 'outsider' (in the past, a minister of religion might have been the right person), or something new, like skilled counselling alongside (and sustaining) the technical, operational business of doing the best for Robert. Neither had been available. On the other hand, the number of highly skilled professionals they had seen come and go over the years (including staff turnover as well as changes of direction) might have amounted to about a hundred.

The message in the letter was that Robert's life and theirs was passing, almost being discounted, while they waited for the 'cure' (really *relief*) which would probably never come. Common sense would suggest that keeping an eye and an ear open for something extra special wasn't inconsistent with taking full advantage of what they had, but grief and anger with themselves, with 'the doctors' and with Robert too were obstructing common-sense decisions. Quite apart from not ever being helped to see exactly what they were doing, their hopes still lay in what the doctors might yet come up with.

Sticking with it was what was needed, staying where they were rather than changing direction once again, and working with professional help on long-standing grief. This would be so difficult to get off the ground. While the letter conveyed my thoughts, as a second opinion should, the intention was as said to affirm the authority and responsibility of those already involved with Robert.

A crisper letter, in terms of making more of the clinical diagnosis, might have been preferred. Instead of talking in terms of various handicaps and a sort of job list, another approach might be to say that Robert showed several symptoms of pervasive developmental disorder, with moderate but definite autistic spectrum characteristics, and that the right treatment, demonstrated by many studies, was a combination of specialised education, social skills training and family work. Naming the devil is as important in medicine as it is in exorcism, I mean in terms of confirming that we know precisely what's wrong, what it's called and what to do. However, apart from identifying what I thought was most disabling, my intention was also to identify where I could see the existing potential, skill and willingness for putting things right. This was 'back home' rather than in the clinic. A letter from the expert stating the diagnosis and treatment could undermine what I was trying to encourage, i.e. their expertise rather than mine. Hence the fine balance needed between the consultative and the clinical style of response, which I hoped was expressed about right in the letter, where it might endure longer than what might be recalled from a single session alone.

6 Refusal

Dear Dr Watkins

Re: Barbara Smith, aged 13

Thank you for asking me to see Barbara, whom I saw with her parents yesterday.

The problem as you say is Barbara's anxiety about going to school, which her parents attribute to bullying, and to what they see as the teachers' lack of interest and consequent lack of action about this. Mr Smith was very angry about this, and he told me, quite forcefully, that he wanted something done about it, and thought that a doctor's letter, for example, from me, would make the school do something.[1] He is not a young man, and he told me about some worries he has about his physical health,[2] which he feels is being badly affected by his frustration with the education authorities. He wondered about seeing you for a check-up and I said I thought he should.[3] On the other hand he wanted Barbara to attend school to keep up with her studies while these things were sorted out. Barbara, looking quite upset, kept telling him not to worry so much. Mrs Smith just seemed very sad, and said fairly little, except that she agreed with her husband.

They wanted me to talk to Barbara and then write to the school, and were rather taken aback when I said I thought we should meet again, saying they had told me everything, Mr Smith in particular wondering if I disbelieved them. They left quite upset and disappointed, and implied that they thought it was negligent of me to have spent most of the time seeing them together rather than questioning Barbara.

I agreed that Barbara needs to be heard, but that what Mr Smith and Mrs Smith thought about the situation was important too. Mr Smith did have some good things to say about the school as well, and I found it difficult in this one session to sort out what Barbara's parents felt needed to be changed at the school and what they felt she ought to be able to cope with. Mrs Smith wondered if there was something I could give Barbara to help her confidence.

I can understand why Barbara and her parents are so upset by all this. It is complicated and confusing.[4]

First, I would like to hear about what is going on at the school, and Barbara and her parents have given me permission to speak to her headteacher. Barbara quite likes her form teacher, and I hope I may speak to her too. However, they didn't want me to speak to the educational psychologist, who Mr Smith explained had been involved but wasn't now. I would like to liaise with him, but of course will not do so without the family's agreement, which I hope they will be able to give me when I have explained how I am trying to help.

Second, I would like to see Barbara again[6] and assess how much of the problem is due to her own anxieties and lack of confidence, which seem to have been around for quite some time, even when school isn't an issue (as in the holidays), and how much is caused by the school. I explained to her parents that a child's problem isn't always as straightforward as it seems at first sight, and that there might be both problems at school and problems primarily in Barbara's feelings, but that at this stage I wasn't sure what the trouble was.[4]

I agreed with Mrs Smith who said they didn't know what to do for the best.[5] They agreed this made it difficult for them to help Barbara become more confident.[8] I said the first step would be for me to find out what is happening at the school, the next to have another talk with Barbara about how she sees the problem and what she thinks will help, and then to all meet again to discuss where we've got to. I said I thought this was the right way to proceed, that is, by looking at all the possibilities, and have made another appointment for a week's time, although Mr Smith and Mrs Smith suggested that it would be unnecessary. I hope they will be able to bring John too.[7]

Thank you for agreeing that I send Barbara and her parents a copy of this letter, which sets out the main conclusions of our meeting.[8]

Yours sincerely, etc.

Notes

1 There was quite a lot of muddle here, and I thought it would be more helpful in the long run to set down in the letter some of the key things being said rather than any premature conclusions of mine. I felt that they were in a sense the minutes of a preliminary and rather chaotic meeting.
2 In fact he looked ill, and I was surprised at his age relative to his daughter and his wife. I wanted to acknowledge this as significant, but it didn't feel right to record here my interpretation of his appearance and body language, which was of physical exhaustion and being emotionally drained.
3 He had been told to see the family doctor again if the symptoms ('indigestion') didn't clear up, but he hadn't, even though the symptoms continued. I decided to check that he would go back, and this sentence was a reminder.
4 I wanted to acknowledge as a very definite observation the fact that I didn't know what was going on. This I thought was honest; it gave the family the reason, true as well as legitimate, why I wasn't plunging in with opinions and advice just yet, and established my wish to explore things further. However, I thought it important to choose words that wouldn't come across as suspicious or intrusive, partly out of courtesy, partly because Mr Smith in particular seemed to feel under siege, and partly because I suspected that there was something rather painful going on.
5 These were Mrs Smith's words, acceded to in a rather subdued way by her husband, in contrast to his alternative message that he knew precisely what was wanted – a quick examination of Barbara and a more or less threatening letter from me to the school about bullying.
6 My instinct was that this was primarily a family problem but that at this stage I believed Barbara hadn't been given enough time to say how she saw it, and I thought she should know that this hadn't been forgotten.
7 The meeting was quite a stormy one, though their anger conveyed depressed despair rather than frustration with yet another stubborn 'official'. They didn't want another appointment (Mr Smith angry, Mrs Smith apologetic, Barbara hadn't wanted to come today) but I gave them one anyway, saying that I hoped they would all come along, including John, Barbara's younger brother. They said he was 'the only one who's alright'. I also said that if Dr Watkins agreed, which I thought she would, I would send them a copy of my letter to her.
    I had tried to make the letter businesslike but friendly, and it could be argued that the conciliatory tone was overdone. However, they struck me as being quite needy

people, rather embarrassed by their anger in the session, and, while we would talk about this at the next session, I wanted the letter to convey the sub-theme of constructive hard talking.

8   Whatever emerged, however, I wanted to remind them of their role in helping Barbara to increase her confidence, to counteract somewhat the ideas that it was all up to the school, or all up to me, or that they were at fault and would be blamed. Feeling at fault is not so easily dispelled, but reminding them in the letter of this positive shared task is one way of beginning.

I also wanted to offer them my uncertainty (about the problem) as an alternative, perhaps even as an antidote, to Mr Smith's show of certainty. Barbara knew that neither the problem nor its solution were that simple, and I believed it would help her to know that asking more questions about it, carefully, with outside help, was feasible, worthwhile, and could be more helpful than the quick solution being proposed.

Comments

I wanted to convey that to help Barbara, more needed to be asked about and handled than bullying. Possibly the letter plays down the latter a little too much, and in fact I would ensure that my enquiries at the school would include questions about bullying. Nevertheless, the letter would have confirmed Mr Smith's suspicions that I didn't really think this was the main issue. I suppose I thought that he didn't either.

I also wanted to show them that perhaps there were aspects to the problem that they hadn't thought of, which at one level indicates that there is quite a lot that can be done to help; and at another that the particularly painful, unexamined corners of their distress had been noticed.

I had wondered if Mr Smith, who was quite elderly, might have a serious physical illness, perhaps cancer. He hadn't, but he had hypertension and angina, still ran his business (although it was floundering), was depressed, and regularly lost his temper over business and domestic matters. Everyone, including himself, feared he was going to drop down dead in the middle of a row, as had his father. As his business problems worsened and the family income dropped, his bad temper had become more evident and Barbara's school refusal had begun. A day away from home was agony, in case 'something happened'. The bullying was minor, by Barbara's admission, amounting to transient teasing which she later said she had used as an excuse. Mr and Mrs Smith regarded Barbara's school non-attendance as the last straw, somehow indicating the family's progressive decline as well as attracting alarming official letters from the Education Department to pile up with those from the Inland Revenue. They felt embattled, and I think were helped a little by my letter, which Mr Smith later recalled as representing a sort of balance sheet. Things didn't turn out too badly, Barbara returning to school once Mr Smith had had a thorough check-up, and we discussed the anxieties he had about his age and his father's sudden death.

The letter, which took longer than usual to compose and probably quite some time to read, may have helped shorten therapy. After what was on the face of it an unpromising start, the second session went better, with the problems of being an elderly parent becoming a useful focus, and John contributing very positively. Mr Smith's physical check-up helped considerably. At the end of the final session Mr Smith commented cheerfully: 'You never know how things are going to end.'

7 Diagnosing the treatment

Dear Dr McAdam,

Re: Donald Jones, aged 15

Thank you for asking for my opinion about Donald's diagnosis and treatment.[1] He and his parents wanted to ask me generally about manic depressive illness,[2] too, and I confirmed that this condition is seen from time to time in young people.

I agree that manic depressive illness is the problem, and that lithium treatment, with regular blood checks, is what is needed.[3] Although Donald has been very unwell he has begun to show quite a lot of improvement, and we were able to have a very calm and sensible conversation today.

Donald's parents were quite right to seek some help for the family as a whole, but it's a pity they felt they had to arrange this independently, understanding that the staff at the —— Hospital didn't have the time to provide this.[4] I know they are short staffed and very busy. Family counselling of the sort which helps relatives understand the illness and its treatment, gives practical advice and enables everyone to be calmer and less annoyed with each other can help, and I would recommend it. However, I didn't get the impression that this rather specific approach is the sort of family help Donald and his parents were getting.[5] Rather, they seemed to have got the impression from their therapists, correctly or incorrectly, that the purpose of the sessions was to ventilate strong feelings that they had suppressed. The family have had two sessions, with everyone feeling quite troubled afterwards, and Donald's symptoms sounding worse each time for the next few days. It also seems that the therapists have suggested that the problem is a family one, not a medical problem, and that the family therapy should enable Donald to stop his medication. In my opinion this would be a mistake.

I have seen family or other psychological traumata precipitate manic illnesses in young people, and seen them helped by lithium combined with family work aimed at calming things down. Once recovered, I think there is a place for the exploration of possible sources of stress and strain, and sometimes this can usefully proceed to work with one or other of the family therapy approaches that are available.[5] My concern here, however, is that Donald and his parents are receiving rather different opinions from two different sources, and I cannot imagine such delicate work as combining lithium therapy with family therapy, both effective treatments, being successful unless either a single team does both, or very close liaison is possible between the two sources of advice. Having two different perspectives from two sets of therapists will confuse matters, and, in the present situation, I have the impression of fundamental disagreement about how best to proceed.[6]

Donald's parents approached you for a second opinion because they saw the discrepancy between the two sorts of approach, and were worried, correctly in my view.[7] I think it is important that they let the family therapists know they have sought a second opinion, and why, and that they see Dr Harris before the next family appointment. I'm not sure what the solution is. Possibly Dr Harris' team and the family therapists could find some way of working in close liaison with each other,[8] or alternatively the family work could be taken on by Dr Harris' team. Either way, I imagine Dr Harris would be interested in the family therapists' observations so far, and vice versa.[9] I do want to stress, however, that the most important single thing is that Donald *does* continue with his lithium.[10]

I would like to keep in touch with the situation until it clarifies.[11]

Yours sincerely, etc.

c.c. Mr and Mrs Jones and Donald
     Dr D. Harris, Consultant Psychiatrist, —— Hospital.[12]
     JD and YB, The —— Family Therapy Practice[12]

Notes

1 I wanted to emphasise (by repeating) the specific questions about diagnosis and treatment, the main anxieties here.
2 I wouldn't have used the term *de novo* in a letter if it hadn't come up in the consultation. It has become well known as a diagnosis for adults, but not so much among adolescents, and might have come across as rather heavy. The hospital's letters didn't mention what had been discussed with Donald. We talked about what it meant, generally and for Donald, and I wanted the family doctor to know that I had done so.
3 I thought this needed to be said. Later I said it again.
4 This was quite a big issue which had a direct bearing on Donald's care, and I wanted to acknowledge this reality.
5 Many of these points are about the different things professional workers mean by 'family therapy'; like many people, including some family doctors, Donald and his parents had little information about what each entailed, what the principles were, or that there were a number of different approaches and controversies about both indications and practice. I thought I should expand a little to indicate what I thought was the normal range of options.
6 There are just too many issues here, each one a minefield for Donald's care, but I think the letter opens them up enough. Meanwhile, my point is to state that there seem to be at least three potential differences of opinion between the two sets of

therapists. I would say that this, together with my own view about lithium, are the main points I wanted to make in the letter.

7 At the same time, although I thought the family therapists were wrong about what Donald needed, it would not be right to be dismissive or offensive; indeed, this letter could have been written in a way which they could have regarded as libellous, and their skills and availability could yet help. It is *very* important to be aware of the effects of fantasies and projections about unknown therapists and institutions.

8 As long as I made it clear what I thought was needed, and I think I did, there was nothing lost for Donald and his family and perhaps something to gain by treating the two sets of contenders with equal respect and as continuing potential sources of help.

9 The letter becomes somewhat prescriptive here, tactfully enough I hope. Whoever works with Donald and his family will need to work together. Whether easy, problematic or impossible, that is what is required.

10 As I said, I didn't want this view to risk getting lost in the discussion about the pros and cons of the rest of Donald's care.

11 This final line shows the suppressed bossiness of the rest of the letter becoming less containable. It would have been better, however, to ask Dr McAdam to let me know how things turned out.

12 The copy to the psychiatrist is with the family's knowledge, and to the family therapists with the family's permission.

8 The wrong patient

Dear Dr Makepeace,

Re: Shelley James, aged 12

Thank you for asking me to see Shelley, whom I saw with her parents yesterday. You will have received my message left with your secretary.[1]

Shelley seems to have a lot of worries troubling her, but she found it difficult to go into detail.[2] Her teachers confirm that she had suffered recent problems with concentration and behaviour. She had previously been[3] a lively, sociable and academically quite successful girl.

Shelley's father spoke on behalf of both parents, her mother being somewhat reticent. She made it clear, however, that she was quite critical of Shelley, and relations are clearly troubled between them. This too is a relatively new development.[4]

The interview was rather difficult, everyone seeming very anxious not to hurt someone else's feelings. When I saw Shelley by herself she looked very upset but wasn't able to say why. I decided it might help to have a word[5] with Shelley's mother, by herself, and concluded that she had become severely depressed, probably since the sudden death of her father about a year ago. She was very close to him. She has been very reluctant to seek help, and I know she has not seen you about this problem, feeling, as she says, that you are quite busy enough and that she should be able to pull herself together. She takes a pride in her self-reliance, indeed, as her husband put it, she always puts others first, in the family and outside.[6]

I told her that this wasn't about self-reliance; rather, that she had become quite severely depressed.[7] She is losing weight and not sleeping, and although she is not seriously contemplating self-injury or suicide, she observed that she wouldn't mind if she were dead.[8] She is reluctant to seek psychiatric help in her own right, but she did agree to see you.

I gave Shelley and her parents a provisional appointment for a week's time, but said that I wasn't sure at this stage how best to use it, i.e.primarily for Shelley, for her mother or for the family as a whole. Before making detailed plans I would prefer to keep a close eye on things while we see what emerges from Mrs James' meeting with you.[9]

I will telephone in a day or two.[9]

Yours sincerely, etc.

cc. Mr and Mrs James and Shelley.

Notes

1 For the record, and not strictly necessary. I suppose it made me feel better, since I thought persuading Mrs James to seek some help in her own right was going to be crucial but might be difficult, and I wanted to have on file my attempt to establish direct contact with the practice.
2 It took me a little time to find the best way of describing Shelley's mental state, and it came down to this. It allows for Shelley's problem being not psychiatric at all, but simply a young adolescent's predicament about what to feel and how to respond to a crisis involving her parents.
3 This struck exactly the wrong note. It is too cautious, too clinical. I should have written, colloquially and boldly, 'is normally' lively, sociable, etc.
4 Again, I am sitting on the fence. I wasn't sure then that this was a well-balanced family enjoying good relationships with each other, sailing along happily until torpedoed by the death of Shelley's grandfather and her mother's prolonged and catastrophic reaction. *Of course* one can speculate about this particular family's normal imperfections and adaptations, but not now, nor in this letter.
5 Why not simply say 'I saw Mrs James by herself', and so on? I think I wanted to convey something to Shelley and her father about my uncertainty (or that it needed at this stage to be uncertain) while we hunted, so to speak, for the source of the problem. They were all sharing a predicament, and needed to know they would all be attended to as necessary; but at this stage I didn't want anyone to feel ruled out, or ruled in, by my interim clinical impressions and hence used the colloquialism.
6 As long as Mrs James knew that I was concerned about her health, a reassuring comment that I knew what she was 'really' like, at her best, seemed in order and

kind. But it would have been a mistake to emphasise her strengths if, in the session and in the letter, I had not also demonstrated that I recognised she was in a hole and feeling helpless.

7 I wanted to confirm how depressed – ill – she was, to counteract her anxiety and, conceivably, anyone else's mistaken assumption that there might be more 'deserving cases' than hers. Not wanting to waste people's time, or to be a burden, can be just one of those things people say, or can indicate highly dangerous depths of shame and guilt. It was these words of hers that made me decide to see her by herself, and to establish telephone contact with her GP.

8 This, for Mrs James, was a private feeling that she was embarrassed about her husband and daughter knowing; although she was glad when they did know, and they were relieved when their worst fear, about whether she would be found dead (like the grandfather when he'd had his stroke), was ventilated.

9 As in n. 5, the intention was to convey that help would be available, but not precisely what help it would be, because I didn't yet know. Mrs James' illness was too big a variable to be sure, at this stage, what else would be needed once she was accepting some help, or particularly if she wasn't.

Comments

My assumptions at the stage when this letter was written were (1) that Mrs James had a quite severe depressive illness, and that it was probably sufficiently self-perpetuating to persist with whatever psychotherapeutic help was directed towards its probable aetiology (her relationship with her father and his death) and towards the family; and (2) that the most likely problem driving Shelley's distress was the expectation that it was her responsibility to recognise her mother's problem and to do something about it.

One strategy would have been to use family work to point out that something wasn't working in the family hierarchy – that something about Mrs James' disabled state had also disabled Mr James, leaving Shelley in charge of something that so far couldn't be talked about even by the adults, let alone handled. I believe this might have gone some way towards relieving Shelley's problem, reminding her father of his capacity for action, and ideally leading to her mother getting some help in her own right, perhaps over the next week or two. I think this might have been a reasonable way of proceeding, and consistent with a unitary theory of family psychiatry. However, particularly as Shelley was so young, I thought it would be better to confirm that her mother was indeed unwell and 'needed to see the doctor', probably given a prescription for medication and conceivably (that is, thinkable, if unlikely) admitted to hospital. Talking about it, and the decision about what to talk about, was important, but came second. The adults whom Shelley perceived taking action were myself and her GP, a woman; for a short but crucial time we acted as parental *alter egos*. This came up quite usefully in a later family meeting, bearing a complex relationship with Mrs James' feelings about her father's medical care during his final illness, and how doctors didn't know everything.

9 All about obsessionality

Dear Dr Cartwright,

Re: Felicity Lee, aged 14

As Felicity's parents feel muddled about the conflicting advice they have had about her problems, and as the treatment plan I am suggesting for her includes several quite different approaches,[1] I thought it would be helpful to sum them up in this letter, with a copy for Felicity and her parents.[2]

1   I think the two most important treatments are the medication, paroxetine, and the behaviour therapy programme, which consists largely of response prevention. I think both should continue as at present, but with closer attention to the behaviour therapy whose importance Mr and Mrs Lee hadn't fully appreciated.[3]
2   As part of this tighter supervision, I suggest the self-monitoring chart should be reinstated, preferably with the family completing it every evening, but with Felicity's parents filling it in if she can't keep it up herself.
3   I don't really think the counselling Felicity is having at school will make a difference to her obsessional problems, and as you know her counsellor Mrs —— agrees. However, Felicity finds her supportive, and wants to continue seeing her. My advice, having discussed this with Mrs ——, is for the counselling to be seen *not* as something that will help Felicity with her habits, which it will not, but (a) to provide a place for Felicity to talk about the strong feelings she will undoubtedly have now that the behaviour programme is being pursued firmly at home, and (b) to help her handle her school work until her checking habits improve.[3,4,5]
4   Finally, I think everyone in the family would find it helpful to discuss the difficulties of adhering to the treatment plan, and I suggest this is the focus for family therapy, at least to begin with.[3]

Yours sincerely, etc.

Notes

1   I wanted to widen the reasons why Felicity's treatment plan was falling apart, rather than leaving her parents just feeling to blame.
2   The style of the letter, summing up and spelling out the programme, was primarily for Felicity's and her parents' information. It could as well have been addressed to them with a copy (with a covering note) to Dr Cartwright.
3   There is an attempt – perhaps slightly obsessive? – to give some logical order to a number of treatments that have accumulated somewhat independently.
4   Of course it was professionally necessary as well as a courtesy to discuss a modified

place for counselling with the counsellor, but I thought it was also important to say so in the letter. It would have been a good idea to send a copy to Felicity's counsellor (with permission, because quite apart from the letter being about wider issues than counselling, it is also about Mr and Mrs Lee); even better, to suggest that Felicity discusses it with her counsellor, again with her parents' agreement.

5   'Habits' and 'checking habits' were Felicity's words.

Comments

What's happening here? Treating obsessive-compulsive disorder can sometimes feel like a battle of wills, one super-ego locking horns with another. Response prevention, which had been making some headway, led to family rows which made Felicity's parents feel very uncomfortable, albeit (probably because) they were full of cold anger and silences and the message, conveyed by Felicity, that her parents were being damaging to her in supporting a response prevention approach; though it needs to be affirmed that Felicity agreed to the programme and was desperate for help with her obsessive behaviour. This fluctuating ambiguity and indecisiveness goes with the condition and drives everyone crazy, effectively undoing the treatment.

I have never known it to be helpful to explore the ideas that are part of obsessionality, although it is certainly interesting. Therapist and patient can have endless absorbing philosophical discussions about the nature of the condition. What does seem useful, however, is assistance in handling the feelings *about treatment* and the effects of treatment, and even the effects of improvement. The severely obsessional patient feels in touch with dark forces to do with fate and misfortune, and which are all the more powerful for making no sense at all; Felicity, who had the characteristic sense of dread that awful, incredible things *might* happen if she didn't check and double-check (like cars crashing, or her school work disappearing without trace) did not believe any of this for a moment and wanted the nagging psychic itch *but what if?* to go away. Her parents, themselves obsessive, had trouble being strong enough to do what she wanted them to do – to stop her checking, which was the point of the response prevention programme.

The feelings that needed working with were therefore not the feelings of obsessionality, which were too embedded in the cognitive and behavioural acts themselves to be accessible, but the feelings provoked by doing what everyone knew to be right: stopping the nonsense behaviour. Mr and Mrs Lee had the idea of being firm hopelessly mixed up with being hostile, intrusive and damaging; Felicity knew their uncertainties and felt her symptoms were stronger than her parents' resolve; she would have loved them to have helped her put things right, even taking control if necessary, but what she experienced from them were ineffective attempts at dominance alternating with extreme discomfort, embarrassment and backing off. She learned to trust her own awkward and time-consuming methods in her embattled circumstances, rather than their half-cock dabbling, and *in extremis* just pushed them away. These were the feelings that could be worked with, being not just more accessible but very obvious, indeed sometimes physically expressed, although with pushing and escaping rather than violence and struggling.

What was needed was authority to control the situation and keep it safe, and one way of doing this was with the authority of a consistent plan: that everyone wanted Felicity to stop doing what she does, Felicity more than anybody; hence, stop it. Stopping it causes side-effects – pain, distress, doubts, what if and so on, so Felicity's individual discomfort is to be taken to her counsellor, and the family's battles to the family sessions, while the response prevention (stopping it), like a necessary surgical operation, just carries on. The SSRI (selective serotonin re-uptake inhibitor) medication is likely to help as well, since, through anti-depressant and other effects it seems to help people rise above fears they know to be unnecessary. It had already been started, though my own inclination would have been to get the psychological therapies consistently under way before deciding if the drug was also necessary. The letter, to all concerned, was in effect a letter of authority to proceed.

Perhaps this type of prescriptive letter has another sort of authority too, the magic of the prescription or formula. If you have difficulties with notions of the power of magic, ask the characteristically intelligent, very rational, obsessive person why they do what they do, and pursue their answer a little, if they allow you to. Perhaps what's needed, then, is even stronger magic.

Chapter 5

Work in progress I

Starting, negotiating, renegotiating

---

10   A slight misunderstanding

Dear Sean,[1]

I'm sorry that you were so upset by your visit to see me, and although I would have preferred you to stay and discuss things, I can understand why you decided to just go. Your mother asked me to say, in this letter,[2] that she should have explained to you that I was a psychiatrist, and she wanted me to tell you that she was sorry she told you that you were coming for an X-ray, although I know that by now she will have apologised to you herself. However, she has had her problems too, not knowing what to do for the best about your angriness, and expecting that you'd be furious with her and that you might even hit her if she said she wanted you to see a psychiatrist. She thinks you are unhappy underneath, and she might be right. I don't know, because we haven't had a chance to talk about it, but if she is right that doesn't make you crazy.[3] Anyway, I wanted you to know that psychiatrists see lots of people who are upset or angry about things, sometimes with good reason, sometimes not, but usually when there are misunderstandings and disagreements. We do see quite ill, disturbed people too, in just the same way your own doctor sees ill people as well as people with what I would call 'normal' problems.[4]

I do think your mother got it wrong with what she told you, and as I said I'm not surprised you blew up in the waiting room,[5] but I still think you ought to come along anyway,[6] because your mother really was trying her best to help, and deserves respect for that. So I hope we do meet, sometime.[7]

I have enclosed a stamped envelope if you would like to write back with your own thoughts about all this.[8]

Yours sincerely,

Dr etc.[9]

Notes

1   Sean was only 14 years old, and I could have written to both him and his mother (his father was long absent) but a personal letter seemed right in the circumstances. His mother, with the best of intentions, and driven by anxiety, had got it wrong, and I thought it more likely that I would see Sean without the issue being forced, and on a basis of trust, if I made this letter something between ourselves.
2   However, it was also important to make it clear that his mother wasn't left out, that she was involved in my writing to Sean, that she knew she had been mistaken, but also that there were reasons for this in Sean's behaviour.
3   I do have misgivings about referring to 'madness' or 'craziness'; it isn't just the ambiguity of the colloquialism (the words are variously used in sympathy, despair, in anger, in mockery and sometimes in admiration), but the notion exists that 'real' madness is always a different patient's affliction, or something non-clinical and beyond even psychiatry; that true craziness is always round the next bend. Very ill people, especially when recovering, or with that part of themselves that is intact, will use such words about others. On balance I think the ambiguity is a helpful one. I have seen psychotic people helped in their social skills, among other things, by distinguishing between what is crazy and what is not. I don't think we need to be over-respectful of the symptoms of madness. All of which is simply about pausing for a moment's thought about using the word.
4   These few lines have something of the flavour of a child's guide to psychiatry about them, but on balance I thought they were OK.
5   As mentioned earlier, repetition has its place in these letters; it is about taking the recipient through it again, a reassurance that the problem and the people have been recognised. It is a reminder of the form of the letter, not just its contents; of the importance of the music as well as the words.
6   A little bit of bossiness here, coming up front about the whole purpose of writing. It is also to be expected from someone whom Sean was reluctant to meet, indeed allowing that perhaps he had a point.
7   But, in the end, one can only hope.
8   I thought it unlikely that he would phone, although I have invited some reluctant attenders to do so; I have also occasionally phoned them at home, taking great care with the decision to do so and how, so as not to appear too intrusive. An SAE seemed right here. Sean didn't use it, but was thoughtful enough to return it.
9   I usually sign my letters as on page 24, which, either with first name or initials, is more or less conventional among doctors. (It bears relation to another convention: that on business cards and letterheads one may be John Smith, MB, BS, FRCP, or Dr John Smith, but it is a touch improper to be Dr John Smith, MB, BS, FRCP. My own are slightly improper, as it happens.) Be that as it may, when writing to some young people, either because they are chronologically children or because they are in a childlike role or mode which I want to acknowledge, I sign off, here, as Dr. I left off 'Consultant Psychiatrist'. I didn't want to rub it in, and the letter was substantially about seeing the psychiatrist anyway, so the reality wasn't being denied. Again, it deserved some thought.

Comments

There isn't a lot more to say. This letter was partly about reassurance. Reassurance can be a weak move in psychiatry, and one should take care not to airily dismiss fears that need facing. However, the main fear the letter was designed to deal with was what Sean imagined psychiatry, psychiatrists and psychiatrists' clientele to be like, and whether he wanted any involvement in it. His mother's way of handling his fears and the fact of a psychiatric referral wasn't encouraging. Thus I thought the letter needed to be both properly professional (and professionalism is about safety as well as other things) *and* to appear to come from a human being.

I also thought it important that the letter should acknowledge, without overdoing it, the awkwardness of this first appointment; it had been a mess, the sort of messes great and small in which adolescents find themselves. I didn't want to convey the impression that nothing much had happened; rather, that it had been a mess, and that messes can be cleared up.

11 Boring

Dear Anne

Thank you for your thoughtful letter. I'm sorry you've decided not to see me again,[1, 2] and I do understand that[3] it was difficult to say so at the last appointment, although I must say I thought you did seem unsure about something when we were sorting out the next one.[4]

I think I know what you mean about the sessions becoming boring. I think it takes two to have a boring conversation, with some responsibility for being boring on both sides.[5] However, boring can be interesting in psychiatry,[6] in fact it ought to be, whatever causes it, because it's quite common as a problem, and because we use the word for all sorts of other things which it is difficult to find the right words for, although I think it is interesting to try. Also, I remember, but perhaps you don't, that you used the word boring quite a lot in the first few sessions, as part of the problem you were seeing me for in the first place.[7]

So, all things considered, I still think it might be a good idea to start again. But if it isn't, and it might not be,[8] it shouldn't be because of anyone boring anyone else.[9]

Let me know what you think.[10]

Yours sincerely, etc.

Notes

1　I wanted to acknowledge Anne's *decision*, and the letter ends with the ball in her court, even though the rest of the letter is about my attempt to make her think again.
2　I also wanted to say something nice about her letter, which showed signs of being difficult to write, and which I guessed (though never asked) was the outcome of several attempts.
3　That, not why. *That* is about her decision, *why* about interpretation, and would have been an impertinence.
4　I wanted to confirm that I *had* noticed that she had seemed undecided about something.

5 I thought there was a value in repetitive use of the word boring. It is a mysterious word, a catch-all for all sorts of interesting and elusive states of feeling, including an ambiguous suggestion of something being not interesting. If we let it pass we can miss something useful. By repeating the word (at the risk of boring the reader) over and over again, I was trying to divest it of some of its slipperiness, that which encourages us to let it go. I wanted instead to swat it, to pin it down and suggest it was something worth examining, that it might even be amusing to do so.

6 Interesting, even fascinating for *psychiatry* rather than for psychiatrists; the impersonal note here is deliberate: see Comments, below.

7 A reminder about the clinical nature of our relationship, and one of the cluster of matters that troubled her – feeling bored and boring, about everything and with nearly everybody.

8 On general principles, I wanted to remind Anne about her autonomy in this situation, her responsibility to decide whether to continue with these sessions.

9 However, I also wanted to indicate that 'being boring' wasn't a reason for not continuing.

10 This was a rather tricky letter, full of pitfalls and allusions (see Comments, below) and I wanted to end on a businesslike note.

Comments

Anne was in psychotherapy, and this letter and the decision that led to it came about a quarter of the way through. She was an extremely intelligent, academic young woman, suddenly going downhill in her work and social relationships towards the end of her first year in university. She was also highly articulate,very mature in manner, almost middle-aged in style, and very serious.

The letter is deliberately playful, a little teasing, although I think it stops short of being flirtatious. I thought about its place on that spectrum with some care, and hoped I'd got it right, which included it being personal but not intimate. I was trying to address both the younger child and the precocious adult in her personality, which had a counterbalancing function: neither was quite right, just like the letter.

In fact she thought the letter was silly. She told me off about it (literature was her subject), ending up amused by her own sternness. I hadn't intended it to be either silly or funny, but I was aware that it was a touch quirky, and this felt OK – a quirky approach to a quirky problem.

I was quite worried about her. She had gone downhill fast, becoming practically socially and academically disabled. She said she felt like a crashed computer. She seemed depressed, but denied sadness, guilt or any of the feelings associated with depression, apart from feeling easily bored and becoming a bore. There were issues in her background, including very high family aspirations and achievement and perfectionism, which made this the likely diagnosis, especially at this particular time – getting *precisely* where she wanted to be, even the specific college. For her problem, whatever it was, she wanted psychotherapy, not medication.

She also had trouble thinking, concentrating and remembering to an extent which led me to arrange for psychological testing and a brain scan: I wondered if she had an early dementing illness, and the first set of psychological tests did not reassure me.

In fact things eventually turned out alright.

12 A problem of persistence

Dear Mr and Mrs Castle,[1]

I wanted to write to you following our discussion at the clinic because I felt you weren't convinced[2] by what I had said, although you did say you were going to press on with the bell and pad for Jack, at least for a time. I'm not surprised that you're wondering whether you ought to seek another opinion, and have never known doctors to be in any way offended by their patients getting another opinion, contrary to what some people think.[3]

I know it was a disappointment after that long session, going over the ground you have all been over before, to end up with the same treatment; indeed, less treatment in a way, because my advice is to give the bell and pad another try but without the night-time medication.[4,5] The problem is that despite all those months of trying, and the similar efforts you all made last year, I am still not sure that this particular treatment has been given a really adequate try.[5] I tried to explain why in the session.

Briefly, I think it should be persisted with. We have to ensure the buzzer can wake Jack, and it would help if he knew you were confident about making it work. Of course you have been frank about your doubts, and I think Sarah —— and I should discuss again with you how the system works, and answer your questions.[5]

I think we can help if we persevere.[6]

I hope therefore that you will keep the next appointment, when we can discuss this again.

Yours sincerely, etc.

c.c. Dr Patel

Notes

1   Jack was quite young (9) and, while one could have written to the whole family, the message in the letter was really directed to his parents.
2   I expanded a little on their doubts about what we were offering, because their non-verbal behaviour towards the end of the session and when we made the next appointment made it clear that they weren't hearing from me what they wanted.

3 Some patients and parents are embarrassed about even wondering about second opinions, and some suspect that doctors will close ranks against them, refuse them all help and so on. I have never come across such attitudes, even in 'canteen culture' conversations. However, I do believe that we have a task, albeit not an easy one, to show we want to stick with patients through difficult times, including doubts and opposition, yet at the same time not making it awkward for them to enquire elsewhere.

4 Medication was an important issue, and seemed to represent for Mr and Mrs Castle treatment that would be entirely a matter for the doctor, rather than something (the night alarm, or bell and pad) which required a plan shared between all. I think I might have put them off by reiterating here what I had been fairly firm about in the session, namely persisting with the behavioural strategy. The clear message about what I was advising and what I was advising against, together with the reasonably clear message that this was going to be something for which Jack's parents should share responsibility, could however have been taken too much as a message to 'take it or leave it'.

5 *Especially* as they were wondering about seeking a second opinion, I thought I should make clear what our own recommendations were.

6 In the session itself, though it was not spelled out in the letter, my co-worker and I had tried to look at their feelings of lack of trust and confidence and the assumption that 'someone' (Jack, themselves, a succession of doctors and psychologists) was necessarily to blame, or not good enough. They weren't happy about our looking at the problem from this wider perspective however, and would have known that continuing like this was part of how we were trying to help.

Comments

They didn't return. Previous specialists had offered medication alone, the bell and pad plus medication, or family therapy, and 'nothing had helped'. The letter was a failed attempt to sustain family work with behaviour therapy as the focus. They returned to the team who had offered medication plus the night alarm, possibly achieving more motivation (having found that the grass wasn't greener in the next field), because this time there was some progress, at least in the short term.

Although it was an attempt to clarify the situation, the letter might have forced the issue, and I think I misjudged their floating the idea of a second opinion, not recognising in their insistence on being in control a wish to be told what to do. It might have been better in this case to confine the letter writing to reminding the family about appointments.

The night alarm has the highest success rate for enuresis, as long as instructions are clear (and correct), properly followed, and persisted with. Unfortunately, particularly where there are wider problems in child and family, pessimism about progress (and attendant apathy) can set in after a series of initial failures.

A better letter might have been as follows.

13 Another attempt

Dear Mr and Mrs Castle,

Following our session yesterday, I thought I should write to acknowledge your doubts about my advice, as I felt that you might decide against keeping the next appointment. I do understand your uncertainty about the conflicting recommendations for Jack's treatment, and your disappointment with the advice you have been given, including my own. If you do decide to come along[1] I will be happy to explain again about the options for treatment available,[2] if that could be helpful, and of course try to answer any other questions.[3] If you don't come, even though I know I advised against seeking *too* many second opinions, I feel the need for Jack to get some help with his bed wetting remains important.[4] Although bed wetting is not the most serious of psychological problems, it can be indicative of other worries that need some help, and in any case Jack will be a much happier, more confident boy once the problem is treated effectively.[5] So do have a word about all this with Dr Patel, and if I don't see you I'll drop a line to him inviting him to give me a ring if he isn't sure who else is available in this field.[6]

Yours sincerely, etc.

Notes

1 This leaves the door ajar rather than closed.
2 In practice, psychiatry is full of contradictions about what needs to be done for whom, even when the research evidence suggests clear enough guidance about how to proceed.
3 Hence an offer of further explanation. The educative role is important in clinical and therapeutic work, and I think more could be made of it.
4 There *is* a problem here; as mentioned above, second opinions are valuable, and in any case patients have no less a natural right to seek them than to obtain estimates from more than one plumber. But second-opinion seeking can also become an unproductive search while the childhood years slip by and potentially useful sources of help are missed. Hence the dilemma is acknowledged here.
5 All of this needs to be said. It would be wrong to prognosticate gloomily about dire consequences, but irresponsible not to remind Jack's parents that this is a serious matter if not a serious 'disease'.
6 Here the family are, as it were, reconnected to their family doctor if, as suspected, they disconnect from my clinic. They shouldn't be left high and dry.

Further comments

We value our opinions, but our clientele may not. While everyone remembers the awkward patient, most patients and families treat therapists with courtesy and respect, and don't always tell us if what we propose or attempt seems unhelpful. We should explore why, not only in terms of feelings but in terms of whether we have explained the situation sufficiently. The notion of the patient as customer conveys something of the new managerial jargon that grates, yet the new perspective it proposes of the doctor–patient relationship may be valuable.

14 Drugs update

Dear Mrs Harris,[1]

You were quite right to call my secretary about running out of David's medication, and I enclose another prescription for just a few days' supply. I am delighted to hear how well he has done, but I do think you should continue to keep the appointments here for the time being, and press on with the behaviour chart, despite the vast improvement.[2]

I enclose another appointment. Please let my secretary know if it isn't convenient.

Thank you also for the newspaper cuttings and printouts.[3]

Yours sincerely, etc.

Notes

1 Again, it seemed right to address the letter about this quite young boy to his mother, rather than to both of them, since we (the clinic) were working entirely with Mrs Harris' authority, and I believe there was nothing special to communicate to David. To the extent that his mother may be misunderstanding or misusing the clinic's advice (about attention deficit hyperactivity disorder in this case), this needs to be talked about with David present, for reasons discussed below, but in a session, not a letter.
2 Dramatic progress *can* happen in child and adolescent psychiatry, and the practitioner need not be incredulous. I believe a level acknowledgement of David's progress with a reminder that the job isn't finished is appropriate, as is the rather controlling decision to provide only minimum medication.
3 Such news about the latest research in one's field, or versions of it, produces mixed feelings, but is generally helpful one way or another. One should always say 'thank you'.

Comments

Despite years of controversy there is still some uncertainty about the place of stimulant drugs such as methylphenidate (Ritalin) in the treatment of attention deficit hyperactivity disorder (ADHD). In the UK and Europe the usual approach to children with conduct disorders which include overactivity is to combine family therapeutic, behavioural and educational strategies, adding methylamphetamine or similar medication to that programme if there is no progress, if progress levels off leaving persisting problems, and if the boy's or girl's state is sufficiently like

ADHD. The accumulating evidence does suggest that methylamphetamine makes a difference to many children regardless of the other treatments, and in North America, clinical practice tends to recommend a trial of medication early on (e.g. a review by Swanson *et al.*, 1998). However, there is a place for clinical judgement, clinical instinct and informed family preference alongside the data of evidence-based medicine; the appearances of ADHD merge on the symptom spectrum with the appearances of conduct disorder (that is, in terms of what you find in clinical assessment, whatever the psychopathophysiology beneath), and similarly conduct disorder merges imperceptibly with normal misbehaviour. Moreover, medication has its psychological and physical problems and dangers. I thought it important that someone should keep an eye on David, keep afloat the other common-sense strategies for his upbringing, and monitor his progress, while trying not to diminish the family's delight at his improvement and their proper and healthy impatience to leave child psychiatry behind.

15 Can't carry on like this

Dear Mr and Mrs Moss, Laura and Andrew,

I wanted to confirm some of the conclusions I believe we reached yesterday.[1] I know it was a very difficult session.

First, I have no doubt at all about the extremely painful and difficult situation at home.[2] Andrew is behaving in ways you disapprove of, and which upset everyone, especially Laura. I don't believe Andrew is happy with how things are turning out either.[3] You also fear that Andrew is risking a clash with the law in some of his behaviour, and perhaps putting himself at serious risk in other ways too, but, as I have seen for myself, he seems unable or unwilling to reassure you other than by saying that he can look after himself.[3, 4]

Having acknowledged this, however, I have to tell you that in my opinion Andrew is not suffering from a psychiatric disorder. That's not to say that he has no problems, or that you have no problems with him.[5] If he wanted help of a psychological or psychotherapeutic nature this should be offered, either here or, because of Andrew's age,[8] at a clinic or centre for young adults. But he has made it clear he doesn't want help and says very strongly and clearly that he doesn't need it.[5]

I know you were very angry, Mr and Mrs Moss, that exploring all the options included pointing out Andrew's right to refuse treatment;[6, 8, 9] and that you felt you had made some real progress by persuading him that he had to come along to the clinic or you would have made enquiries with the social services or with your lawyer if he had refused.[9] I think you are both absolutely right to see the problem in legal and social terms, and there is every reason why you should pursue that course if necessary. In fact I regard your warning that you will call the police if there is further violence, or any other activity in your home[10] that you object to, perfectly reasonable, in Andrew's interests, and not at all extreme. Of course, Andrew, part of the process of any legal action would mean having your own views fully represented from the start.[7]

I sympathise with your request, Mrs Moss, to have some further appointments here by way, as you say, of support and keeping an eye on things.[11] We have been doing this, I think, and it has been valuable in clarifying what is happening at home and what can and cannot be done about it. It has been important for me to meet Andrew, and to reach some conclusions about his mental state and his plans and wishes. However, I believe we have reached a point where further support will mean reinforcing an intolerable situation and perpetuating it, perhaps even making it worse, while simply hoping that something will change.

I am sorry to say however to all of you that I don't think things will change as long as the argument is around whether or not psychiatry can help, and that the short-term alternatives open to you all are the legal or social ones we have discussed.[12]

If Andrew were to choose to ask for some personal help, that would be a completely new situation, and I would be very happy to talk to him about it. As we agreed, I have sent a copy of this letter to your family doctor.[13]

Yours sincerely, etc.

Notes

1 Everything in this letter was discussed in the session referred to, its tone throughout being to deliberately confirm what was said.
2 Andrew is behaving abominably, but nevertheless an objective statement about the situation seemed the firmest basis from which to try to effect change. Andrew can dispute 'being' bad, and does, bringing in accusations about his parents' present and past behaviour in order to question who is also 'bad'. This is one of many ways in which the family arguments go round in circles. He cannot, however, deny that his parents disapprove, or that Laura is upset by him.
3 This refers to another important family dynamic: Andrew doesn't mind that his family believe he is moving in wild circles and putting himself at risk. On the other hand, I didn't believe he was entirely happy with the situation.
4 I could have written that Andrew is stealing, making use of stolen goods and taking illicit drugs, among other things. These are the sorts of things his parents suspect and fear, and Andrew allows them to. Again, the known facts are only the fears which Andrew encourages, and I think it would be wrong, even in a confidential letter, to state that he is being delinquent.
5 It is important to acknowledge the size of the problem, even though it isn't of a psychiatric nature. People can believe very strongly that, by default, any problem not amenable to another remedy is by definition psychiatric. If that is what is seriously believed, I think psychiatrists should show an interest, but they should

also be prepared to explain if psychiatry isn't indicated, or (as in this case) wouldn't work without the potential patient's co-operation.

6 In writing this letter I might have been carried away into an absorbing debate about the place of compulsory treatment, but it didn't arise in the session; this in itself was interesting. I don't believe Andrew's parents thought that he was 'mad', even though at the first session they had asked (and been told) about schizophrenia. They saw Andrew's behaviour as representing a 'split personality', which even many well-informed people equate with schizophrenia. (It provided an opportunity to talk about his sensible, thoughtful side.)

7 This point is pivotal. One of Andrew's constant and angry complaints is that, far from being crazy, he simply isn't being listened to. On the other hand, the situation has reached the point where listening to each other isn't feasible whether in the clinic or at home.

8 A reminder about his age – nearly 20 – and legal autonomy.

9 Andrew's parents had shown resourcefulness in the way they had persuaded him to attend a second session, and had used their own authority albeit talking vaguely about what he would 'have' to do or they would 'damned well do something about it'. They also, unusually, acted very much together, and made it clear it was also to help Laura, and because they thought Andrew needed help too. All this was commendable, but 'nearly but not quite', because it was done in an eruption of firmness which they couldn't sustain. They deserved encouragement, but also the reminder to 'now do it properly', which would either be family therapy (with Andrew agreeing to participate) or taking legal action. But *apart* from the dynamics of the case, Andrew needed to know his rights in this situation too, not only as a matter of ethics and law, but because being dead straight with him was crucial as a basis for any eventual development, whether it was legal, social or therapeutic.

10 I nearly used 'in your own home' here, with all the indignation on the parents' behalf which the phrase contains. However, it was still Andrew's home too, despite his abuse of it. I thought it would be better to include a gentle reminder that his parents should decide what is acceptable at home. Andrew wasn't an intruder; the problem was that he wasn't being helped towards independence. If he was outstaying his welcome, his parents needed to find a way to say so other than pleading insanity on his behalf.

11 Mr and Mrs Moss were very persuasive on this point, and I could well have seen them once or twice more, or indeed once or twice too often. Andrew had only come to the first session, and this second one, under protest. But I believed the side-effects as described in this paragraph were making things worse, which is also why the case differs from Letter 3.

12 I thought a longish letter was more likely to be read thoughtfully, at least by Andrew's parents, than a short one. They had worried and ruminated about Andrew for ages, and the letter was designed to match the drawn-out, repetitive nature of the problem. Mr Moss, I knew, would have gone through it carefully, making pencilled annotations. But it had to be summed up briefly, hence this penultimate paragraph.

13 But I thought it important to state this too, especially as it might have been a surprise in the tail end of the letter. It wasn't inconsistent with the message preceeding it, although I did wonder if the parents might have spied with relief a

chance, however illusory, to procrastinate with 'one more try'; hence I reminded them how novel it would be if Andrew asked for help for himself. However, another therapist might well have decided to end the letter at the previous paragraph.

Comments

The importance of establishing authority and consent for therapy cannot be overestimated, not only because of the obvious legal and ethical implications but to make therapeutic work feasible and sustainable (Steinberg, 1987, 1992a). This is true, I believe, in all fields (how much medical advice and medicine isn't taken properly because it doesn't have *the patient's* understanding and conviction?) but it is particularly true, and particularly elusive, in work with young people, where authority and responsibility are unpredictably and sometimes chaotically distributed between family members, school, various therapists and helpers, real or imagined cultural expectations and the many shades of grey in the law.

There was a clear family dynamic operating in this family's case, and an alternative view could be to battle on, bringing the various issues raised in the letter into the sessions as items for the agenda. To this extent a letter like this could be brought along as the basis for a family contract, and helping the family turn it into one as a therapeutic strategy. My own conclusion was that matters were going to go downhill in this family faster than therapeutic work could repair them, that the law would soon be involved in one form or other, and that it would be best if this happened before any more damage was done. Again, I thought that the contents of the letter could be the basis for a court report, suitably rephrased, as much as for a therapeutic contract. Therapeutic work would have depended on the presence of Andrew in body and spirit, and neither could be relied upon.

In the event, non-psychiatric measures (social and housing services and vocational training) resolved everything.

Chapter 6

Work in progress II
General maintenance

---

16 Eleven years

Dear Dr Blake,[1]

I know you have recently become the above patient's general practitioner, and I thought I should write to you about my work with him, particularly since it goes back such a long way. I have actually been seeing him for eleven years, which is very unusual for me,[2] although our present contact is now, by agreement, only three or four times per year, and will probably be less next year.[3]

Mr Allan was first referred to me when he was going through a period of considerable stress in his work (for the Inland Revenue) during the time of his father's last illness. He was then aged 32, and still living at home. He had begun to drink heavily, abuse drugs in a relatively minor, isolated way, was very overweight and was already a heavy smoker. A little later, on my advice, he saw Dr —— for his drug dependence and obesity, and had quite a difficult time during a short admission to his unit, though to the best of my knowledge he has touched neither alcohol nor illicit drugs since. He then had a coronary, fortunately not too severe, on his fortieth birthday, and you will know about his subsequent care at —— Hospital. Since then he has given up smoking completely and watches his diet and weight sensibly.

In physical terms he has made a good recovery, he has progressed steadily in his career, enjoys his hobbies and apart from having relatively few close friends – I should say no intimate friends – he is emotionally stable if a little shy, and is enjoying life, albeit (as he points out) without alcohol, cigarettes and and many 'forbidden' foods, and has no sex life to speak of. He has remained unmarried, although he has had a few girl-friends for short periods.[4]

I should say – and Martin[6] understands – that the period when I was treating him with psychotherapy is behind us. Nor does he want help with any of his minor residual anxieties. He says however that it helps him a lot to see me occasionally, when we have what I suppose I would describe as essentially a psychodynamically informed conversation. He says he has no one else to chat to freely about his thoughts and feelings, as others can with close friends or at the pub;[5] and when we review his contact with me, as I've felt bound to do[7] once a year or so, he says he wishes to continue, yet with no qualms about the intervals between appointments steadily widening. My judgement is to trust him on this point, and I am happy to continue offering him appointments, and will assume this meets with your approval.

I have sent Mr Allan a copy of this letter.[8]

Yours sincerely, etc.

Notes

1 This is an example of a letter which it seemed best to send to the doctor with a copy to the patient.
2 This was a very long period for my usual practice, and I thought it should be put on the table, so to speak, between the three of us.
3 Mr Allan was winding things down at his own pace, and I wanted to acknowledge this for his encouragement, his new doctor's information and for my own treatment plan.
4 The letter would have been too long, and served a different purpose, had I gone into Mr Allan's family background and relationships, and what we had and hadn't dealt with in psychotherapy. The purpose of the letter was to outline his physical and psychiatric history and the nature of his contact with me, and to explain, or justify, my slightly unusual supportive role.
5 I could have used more technical language here, and in fact have largely adopted Mr Allan's style of self-description. Again, this felt right, because of the nature of the letter and its message: the reasons for continuing to see a largely recovered patient. I wanted to convey this in the letter's style.
6 I had used the patient's first name automatically at this point, but not elsewhere. I think the formality/informality ratio probably reflects fairly accurately the formality/informality balance of the professional relationship, and the inconsistency mirrors the ambiguity. I mention this for interest, rather than as a weighty point.
7 Indicating my uncertainties about continuing to see him.
8 It is a letter which, for Mr Allan, spanned some important years and generations, and summed up some key events, however superficially and incompletely. That it doesn't touch on everything is also important: it is an outline of a primarily medical narrative yet one which has been rather central to his life.

Comments

There are some psychotherapists who see people for as long or longer, and perhaps for more subtle problems, who would not find the lengthy story of this man's treatment remarkable. On the other hand my own preference and philosophy favours minimalist interventions, particularly for the younger people who make up much of my work, and eleven years seemed rather long, and needed, I thought, review and the family doctor's approval. Yet the current and anticipated time allotted for treatment *was* pretty minimalist, and I thought had a useful preventive function. I might have spelled this out.

I think I was offering Mr Allan the rather old-fashioned service of the physician/psychiatrist as guide, philosopher and friend, and that in view of his past history – he had gazed into the abyss several times – our contract was a reasonable and indeed economic one.

The point of the letter was that this contract needed to be reviewed and renewed at intervals, a touch on the tiller so to speak to keep the roles, boundaries and work on course. Reminding Mr Allan and informing his GP that I was a specialist seeing him for specific reasons and technically on behalf of his general practitioner, also reinforced what I think is a valuable clinical tradition and an important experience for clinicians outside general practice.

17 A thank you note

Dear Elizabeth,

Thank you very much for the really lovely picture. It must have taken you hours. I recognised Boris and Floppy straight away. You must be enjoying school once again, which is very good news. Well done.

Thank you again, and best wishes for the future.

Yours sincerely,

Dr D. Steinberg

Comments

I didn't think this letter needed annotations. I didn't want it to be too long, which would have made too much of a post-treatment contact and in any case would have been unnecessary; nor too short, which might have come across as perfunctory. I recognised the pets in Elizabeth's drawing, but had to check the notes to make sure I got their names right.

As I said earlier, I think signing as Dr (or even Doctor) is the proper usage for a letter to a child or young adolescent, though I wouldn't specify an age. You will know which is right as long as it crosses your mind, which it should.

18 No more letters please!

Dear Mr Smythe,[1]

What a lot of questions![2] You do raise points which as you say require my response, but they seem to me very much the sort of thing we all discuss anyway when we meet.[3] I think corresponding about them will duplicate matters, and might risk becoming a diversion and distraction too.[4] I will save up your faxes and letters for our next appointment,[5] and, of course, make sure they are on our agenda. However, I would prefer it if you stopped sending any more for the moment.

With kind regards,[6]

Yours sincerely, etc.

Notes

1   The length of this letter is important. It could have been half as long but, as I said for Letter 17, it would have seemed curt. As it was, Mr Smythe thought it brusque.
2   I didn't particularly like this expression, and I can't think of another time I've put it in a letter. It conveys the jolliness of the *really* irritated and is also patronising, in a way which might be alright if diluted in the to and fro of conversation. It is probably effective as a cause for pause, but on paper it risks perpetuating mutual antagonism. I used it after some thought about the recipient, whose pomposity and 'busy-ness' was not only rooted in his anxieties, but also related directly to the problems for which I was seeing his son, in which a rather obsessive intrusiveness was a factor.
3   If the first two points sound like arm-wrestling on paper, and therefore somewhat manipulative, albeit with therapeutic intent, *this* point is transparently straight and true. Everything Mr Smythe was pressing me on was central to what we needed to talk about together, preferably in the family meetings (see Comments, below).
4   This too was accurate. I predicted that he would enquire, 'Distraction from what?'
5   This point served a number of purposes. Mr Smythe's letters and the fax which preceded each were long and clearly treasured, with the legalistic phrasing lengthy, obsessive and finely honed. In practical terms it was proper to treat his correspondence with respect, even if I didn't agree to use it as he required, which included demands for immediate replies. However, it enabled me to indicate that the letters would be handled as 'evidence', collated and conveyed to the proper setting, and not ignored. I would place them on the desk when we met.
6   You don't know how a letter will be read. Letters are read aloud, so to speak, with the inner ear listening, and an actor could read the same material in a light or menacing, friendly or unfriendly way. The perceptive reader might have suspected that I found Mr Smythe a little irritating, and while I hope my reply conveyed this in a way which was appropriate and courteous, the closing salutation was intended to confirm that, in the end, things were OK.

Comments

Mr Smythe was an obsessive man, trapped by his efforts to ensure the best for everybody in the most controlling, repetitive and intrusive ways. Of course, this was completely counterproductive, and alienated those closest to him as much as it did his colleagues and acquaintances. It came to a head when his eldest son rebelled, an event which astonished Mr Smythe and shook him badly.

He was also incredulous at the emerging hypothesis that he was a controlling, dominating, aggressive man, though he was also fearful of damaging others or driving them away. This could not have been more different from how he saw himself: mild, nice and put upon. I saw our brief correspondence as complementing what we were trying to deal with individually (with him) and in the family work, not as a supplement to therapy but consistent with it: to demonstrate that antagonism was an issue. It helped that he began to see the funny side of the mounting correspondence on my desk.

19 Well organised chaos

Dear Mr and Mrs Kay, Lucy, Daniel, Anthony and Sarah,

Thank you for your further messages to Ms —— and to my secretary.[1] I can see how difficult it is for everyone to get together to confirm and then keep our appointments. When we discussed whether you really wanted to come along, you told us you wanted to, and that it was important.[2, 3] My impression from what you say is that it is.[4] Could I suggest that rather than Ms —— and I offering another time which in the end you might not be able to make, instead you find a time when everyone at home is together, hold a meeting of your own, and work out say two or three dates which would definitely suit everyone, and drop my secretary a line listing them?[5] Would you do this?[6]

Yours sincerely,

S.M., D.S.[7]

Notes

1 There was a lot going on, with phone calls (from public boxes, with the money running out), faxes from Mr Kay at various airports, and appointments earnestly made and remade, mostly to the team secretary, with messages often left late at night with the in-patient unit.
2 So far – because I really wasn't sure, and I wanted to say that at least one more meeting with everybody was going to be needed to see whether the family felt the effort required was justified by their perception of the problem. The letter from the family doctor was instructive in this respect; he knew them moderately well, mostly via the children, and said that Mrs Kay had asked for the appointment because she was worried about the academic performance of the two eldest children at school. School reports expressed surprise that we were seeing them (in so far as we were), and said there were no anxieties at all about them.
3 However, we didn't send copies of the letter to the family doctor or the school because at this stage we still felt that the letter was in a sense strategic and part of our odd, partial engagement with the family rather than simply something 'for information'. (Had we wanted to send a copy of this letter to the school, we would have sought permission to do so.)
4 I addressed this point to the whole family, while it could have been addressed to Mrs Kay, who initiated the referral and acted as spokeswoman on the only occasion

when we saw them and who was the only proponent of the view that the clinic's help was needed. We thought the question should be addressed to all, however, as we had tried to address it to all in the session.

5 The advice was to get together as a family to make a decision. We gathered this would be something that was (1) welcome, (2) difficult, and (3) unusual. We thought it would help, though not quite in the way it turned out.

6 Persuasive, if not pleading, I hoped, rather than imperative.

7 Elsewhere I have mentioned my own preference for the clinician leading the therapy to sign the letter, rather than having several signatories (p. 28). Here, though, we felt particularly like two teams getting into position for some sort of game, and both my co-worker and I signed.

Comments

We never saw them again. A cancellation message was left with the ward. However, a couple of weeks later a rather nice card arrived, signed, surprisingly, by everyone, with thanks and the message that everything was now fine. They didn't mention whether they had actually met as suggested, so we wrote to ask. We were curious, and not hopeful about a reply; I wanted to enclose a stamped, addressed envelope, but my co-worker thought it would be more informative not to. Mr and Mrs Kay wrote back with a letter they had both signed to say that they had found their meeting at home helpful, and had decided they didn't need to see us after all.

We did let the school and family doctor know that we weren't seeing them, after the cancellation message, inviting further contact if there was any concern. We could have written to the family once again; but in retrospect I think it was right that we didn't, since it seemed that its energies were now better focussed.

20 Keeping channels open

Dear Sue,

Thank you for your note. Jacquie and I have discussed very carefully the message your friend brought, and we think we understand your reasons for not wanting to come again,[1] but we both think you would be making a mistake.[2] Please phone either of us, or Ken, to talk it over.[3] We will do our best to make sure you get through easily.[4] In any case, Jacquie was planning to visit you and the children at home, and will call at 11 on Friday morning, 27th.[5] Please remember our advice to call the police if necessary.[6]

Yours sincerely, etc.

Notes

1 This phrase is an attempt to be truthful enough but not provocative or too anxiety-provoking in what was an exposed and threatening situation. (see Comments, below).

2 For similar reasons it seemed right, and safer, that we at the clinic should be seen to be taking the initiative.
3 Again, this is an imperative statement, albeit framed as a request.
4 This, as well as being realistic about switchboards, confirms that we are taking responsibility for maintaining contact.
5 The message is that a routine visit was planned anyway.
6 A reminder of our advice to Sue.

Comments

This letter needed to be clear and straightforward, yet as far as possible it was important that it didn't make matters worse if read by her boyfriend, an immature, demanding, and intermittently drunk and threatening man.

The circumstances here were complex and not necessarily as they might seem at first sight. In terms of physical violence, albeit not too damaging so far, the worst of it came from Sue, and was generally the way in which an hour or two of drunken, tearful threats and abuse from her boyfriend would be brought to an end.

Sue had been referred, after some hesitation, by her health visitor (who was concerned about the children). Sue seemed to find the session she attended with the children helpful, was pleased to make a further appointment, but then left a message cancelling it. One of us called back, and she said that her boyfriend had warned her not to attend, but that in any case she didn't really want to; she now felt she could handle things and would get back in touch if necessary.

There was some ambiguity in saying that we 'thought' we understood why Sue didn't want to come again, the ambiguity reflecting the truth. Yet the fact that we weren't quite sure, and were prepared to say so, didn't inhibit us from giving five separate pieces of advice in a six-line letter about maintaining contact. This too reflected the situation, where the degree of intervention justified was far from clear, and the task was to keep the channels open in both directions while we tried to see what was needed for whom, what was acceptable, and what (if anything) needed to be forced, meanwhile not making matters worse. The 'message' was that all this sounded worrying and we were taking it seriously, whatever her changes of mind and whatever her reasons. At another level it was about adopting a parental and authoritarian role with a family which consisted entirely of children and people acting like children.

21 Wet blanket

Dear Jason,[1]

I know how reluctant you were to come to see us, and how pleased you must be that the chart and the night alarm are working so effectively. The latest report from school is very good too, as you know. However, despite all this progress[2] I still think you should continue coming here for the family meetings.

When we first talked about this together, you did explain that you appreciated some help with the wetting at night and the soiling, even though I remember you were still very angry with your parents about bringing you along.[3] I also remember that there was a lot of disagreement about the arguments at home, that you felt that your parents were making too much fuss about them, and exaggerating. My impression is that the chart and the night alarm are certainly helping you put part of the problem right, but that the rows still need some more attention.[3] I realise your mother and father think[4] this more than you do. I think the 'arguments' bit of the problem needs the family meetings for three reasons. First, because I think they help your parents even if you don't think they help you, and you are needed to make the sessions useful.[5] Second, because I think the arguments are connected with the other problems, even if you don't.[6] Third, because I think there's a chance that if we can help sort out the causes of all the arguments it will help you manage permanently without the night alarm and the chart, and put things right properly.[7]

I also enclose a copy of the letter I said I would write to your doctor.[8]

Could you discuss both letters with mum and dad?

Yours sincerely, etc.

Notes

1 This could have been written as a letter to the family as a whole, but we were still negotiating how to handle the family rows which everyone knew only too well about, and Jason's encopresis, which he was reluctant to have brought up in front of his younger sister. Writing a letter to the family and not mentioning the encopresis would have defeated the object of writing at all, which was to make a connection between Jason's soiling and wetting and the arguments. So we wrote, over my name, to Jason only, inviting him to discuss the letter with his parents.

2 We acknowledged his progress, which was considerable, even though it seemed that the improvement in one area was at the cost of mounting difficulties in terms of the rows.

3 This is part of the story of Jason's attendance. He was practically dragged to the first session, his anger bordering on violence. No previous treatments had been persevered with (they included the methods we recommended once again, which was another source of disappointment and anger, this time on the part of Jason's parents too, in a session that was particularly useful). Jason wanted to manage the chart and night alarm by himself, especially after an explanation, just to him, about how they worked and why he should persevere with them, and doing so effectively raised his self-esteem, confidence and school performance. He valued these separate, rather mechanistic discussions, but acknowledged that the contract included the family meetings. This was a reminder to him.

4 Referring to his parents' disagreement with him rather than what they 'thought' would have been better, and clearer.

5 I was going to write 'make the sessions work', but that would have leaned too much towards Jason's tendency to dominate and control, and getting the fine

adjustment right as we moved from dominance to autonomy was part of the work. I thought this phrasing 'placed' him more appropriately; or, if you like, put him in his place.

6 For the same reason, the experience of friendly if bossy disagreement was good for him.

7 I thought this was likely to be sufficiently true to justify the time and effort put into persevering with this side of the work, even if his parents had judged his behaviour to be manageable. In addition, again with the balance between domination versus autonomy in mind, I thought he was entitled to an account of a hypothesised dynamic which might otherwise have remained a mystery.

8 See Letter 22.

Comments

Jason was a very bright 11-year-old, brought to sessions very unwillingly, but who eventually agreed, initially grudgingly and later with some enthusiasm, to accepting help for his enuresis. His parents saw this problem and the soiling gradually diminishing, but were more concerned about the high levels of tension in the family (for which some very understandable reasons emerged), with everyone being on a short fuse which Jason usually lit. There was disagreement between Jason and his parents about how big a problem this was, and he also found it an embarrassment, like the encopresis. At the time the letter was sent, to supplement a rather muddled session, Jason was saying all was now well, an opinion supported by his self-monitoring chart, but his parents were saying that things were as bad as ever. In this session Jason, very upset, talked about his fears of being thought 'mad', which he related to the angry outbursts, and partly to the encopresis, though not at all to the enuresis. There were family issues about mental illness too. There was a very disturbed paternal grandparent, and this had led to issues of emotional control and fears about anger being very important on one side of the wider family. The difference of opinion about what was important for the sessions became a helpful and relatively safe model for negotiating emotionally loaded disputes. We also added angriness and arguments to the behaviour chart, to be monitored not by Jason alone but by consensus between his parents and himself, with the result that the rows diminished and discussion about them became central to the family work. Meanwhile, we suggested that we write the letter below to the family doctor, with a copy for Jason.

22 A further letter

Dear Dr Kumar,

Further to my recent letter about Jason's progress, one of the other things we have been discussing with him and his family is their worry about how Jason's medical files will record this episode and his contact with us, with particular concern about him being described as mentally ill. There is a related worry about this getting into other computer systems outside the health service.

I would not describe Jason's condition as a mental or psychiatric illness, although he does now agree that the wetting, soiling and very upset feelings are big problems that need some help. Children learn to control their body functions at different rates, some people taking longer than others. If there is a lot of worry and tension in a child and the family, this can result in a habit gained (like bladder and bowel control) being lost for a time, or a delay in acquiring the habit. I think this happened in Jason's case, that he was vulnerable to this sort of physical problem, and pressures in the family triggered it off. I explained that it helps us do research in the whole range of children's problems if we do put these problems in our files under the heading 'psychiatry', but as far as Jason himself is concerned, if in the future he wonders whether or not he was mentally ill, or indeed if anyone asks, my view is that the truthful answer is no.

We thought it would be helpful to have this in Jason's records.

Yours sincerely, etc.

Comments

This was a difficult letter to put together. One issue is confidentiality. I used to think people were unnecessarily alarmed about it being possible for confidential medical data to be leaked or tapped into, but now I am not so sure.

A second issue is the risk of reinforcing the impression that mental illness is shameful. It shouldn't be but it can be; it also depends on what people mean by mental illness, and what they think are its implications. Had Jason had a schizophrenic illness we would have had a different sort of discussion, and I wouldn't have written a letter like the one above. But what if he had been a different sort of child, temperamentally, and had become clinically depressed by the family situation? Would that have been classified as mental illness? Anyway, although the clinical, developmental and philosophical debate will continue, I thought that with his particular battery of problems and worries Jason was entitled to help with his perception of himself and to his privacy, and I believe what I said about his problem was as true as anything else that might have been said.

A more immediately serious issue would have been if a letter like this contributed to a denial of his problems; but if anything I think it made it easier for Jason to acknowledge them.

Nevertheless, I felt very slightly uncertain about the issue generally (hence these lengthy comments), and I hope the reader does too.

23 Still more tests

Dear Dr Turner,[1]

Since her admission Ally has been making really good progress, particularly in the unit school here and in the groups. She is now swallowing food and drink without a naso-gastric tube and can walk about with a nurse or one of the other children lightly holding her arm. Her parents, brother and sister are coming regularly for family meetings, and although they could not at first see the point of them, we have explained that even though we don't understand what's gone wrong for Ally,[2] we do think there should be a regular time when the family[3] and two of our staff, Dr —— and Sarah ——, can discuss changes in Ally's condition as they happen, and to keep everyone equally up to date as we help work out what it's all been about.[4]

The same applies to the continuing physical investigations, some of which were of course initiated in your own department. We have explained to Ally and her family that, while it would be nice to be able to say that all the physical tests are completely clear, so that we could put that query behind us and conclude that this is entirely a psychological problem, we really aren't sure, and of course many problems are a bit of both.[5]

We have explained that we don't suspect any dreadful[6] or dangerous condition, which in any case would have been found by now. But it's just possible that there could still be one of those troublesome problems of the body's chemistry that could keep Ally's condition going, and we didn't want to put off her psychological treatment here while we wait to find out.[7] Our guess is that she will continue to make good progress and that all the physical investigations will turn out to be normal.[8]

One of us will write again.

Yours sincerely, etc.

Notes

1 This letter was to the psychiatrist at the referring unit in a paediatric hospital, and is an example of a letter where it is particularly difficult to serve the needs of clinicians as well as an intelligent but young teenager. We could have composed two different letters, but for this first interim report it seemed a good moment to have the same 'document' for the several experts involved as well as the child and her family.
2 The probable psychological and family formulation was as compelling as some of the neurological assessments seemed initially positive.
3 During a period of considerable clinical uncertainty and family anxiety, we believed that family review meetings, taken by the psychiatric registrar and Ally's key nurse were essential, and we had made plans in terms of staff supervision for

the review meetings to shift into family therapy as the changing diagnostic focus clarified what sort of family work would be needed.

4   The ambiguity and slight optimism in the phrase both reflect the clinical impression at this stage.

5   Colloquialisms can be patronising and inept, and care is needed with them, but I think this phrase at this point is about right.

6   Much the same applies to 'dreadful'. It may not be in the textbooks, but it captures what people feel and say about some feared diseases. The type of words referred to in notes 5 and 6 were the sorts of words that came naturally to child, family and staff in the sessions. They were part of the common language generated by this group of people for this piece of work.

7   There is a hint of impatience here to get on with what we think the work needs to be. This was also an accurate reflection of the feelings of those involved.

8   But guesswork nevertheless.

Comments

Ally presented with multiple paralyses and atypical tremors and dystonias, and as she proceeded through several clinics some atypical though borderline neurological and biochemical findings emerged, as they do. Various prescribed drugs and vaguely recalled developmental disorders in the far reaches of the family contributed to the complexity of the history.

Elsewhere (e.g. Letter 5), the problems of serial second opinions are mentioned. People are entitled to second opinions, but there comes a point where repeated pursuit of a hoped-for 'better' diagnosis or treatment plan risks undermining the benefits of the current management, the patient's confidence, spirits and general well being. The risk of this must be balanced against the risk of 'missing something'. Nor does the tidy rule of the medical textbooks – to diagnose first, 'exclude' physical illness, then treat psychiatrically – actually work in real life, where the difference between theory and practice shows that something is amiss with the theory. To undergraduates, clinical psychiatry can seem catch-all and rather woolly, and clinical neurology the epitome of clear-cut diagnosis. In the actual clinical jungle the balance is considerably redressed.

Our plan was to treat what we could see, which was a complex problem requiring psychological and physical rehabilitation, and to be prepared to repeat investigations. Disorders change over time, particularly in developmental conditions.

The following child's case illustrates similar problems of clinical management and how to explain it.

24 Another way of proceeding

Dear Dr McKay,

I said I would write to sum up where we have got to with Terry's investigations and treatment.[1]

As you know, Mr and Mrs Barker are deeply concerned about a physical condition being missed in Terry's case. His unusual symptoms and some of the test results do remain puzzling. I can understand that they want to put psychiatric help on one side while they pursue physical investigations at ―― Hospital, where the ―― Department has received a lot of very favourable publicity in the newspapers recently.

Terry's tests do indeed show a number of unusual features, although the consensus view of the neurologists, paediatricians and psychiatrists who have seen him is that they do not amount to a definite disorder, and it certainly does not seem similar to any condition that is known[2] to get worse or become dangerous. From our point of view we would rather press on and help Terry with what seem to us his obvious psychological difficulties. Terry's parents feel we should 'get to the bottom of it' first, that is, find out if there is a definite physical illness behind it all. We don't agree about the advisability of continuing in this way.[3] I believe Terry understands his parents' and our disagreement about how best to proceed in his best interests, and does not seem inappropriately bothered[1] by this. Our team are happy to continue doing our best to help.[4]

We have asked them to discuss this with you, and I have sent them a copy of this letter.

Yours sincerely, etc.

Notes

1 Terry had a learning disorder. We wanted him to understand as best he could what was going on between the adults, and the letter reflected what we had very fully discussed more than once with the family. Indeed, we felt that while at one level practical questions of choice were being discussed, at another the parents in particular were working through something very important by proxy – what it was that was 'wrong' with Terry. Terry progressively understood what this was all about (see Comments, below) to, we believed, his increasing advantage.

I used the word 'bothered' near the end of the letter because it was one of Terry's own words; rather a nicely ambivalent one, combining the active with the passive experience of being troubled.

2 'That is known' implies uncertainty, which was the real situation. It touches on the clinical dilemma of being scrupulously truthful and therapeutically confident at the same time. This can be managed by teaching our clientele what we know about the balance of probabilities, the risks of a particular course of action *versus* the risks of alternatives, including the risks of inaction, without it becoming so fascinating an academic diversion that therapeutic needs are lost sight of. It is one of the challenges of evidence-based medicine, and the task is for public education to be a key skill for clinicians.

3 Agreement to disagree was right for Terry and the relationship we had with his parents. It emerged in a wider discussion about how to make sense of their history of repeatedly leaving behind medical teams which had sometimes begun to help.

4   The working relationship we had with Terry's parents was good, and because of (rather than despite) this, a lot of anger was expressed in some sessions, causing some anxiety about how much 'going elsewhere' was a rational choice and how much an angry and rejecting gesture on one side or the other. This surfaced usefully in team meetings too. We tried to make the wording here helpful and friendly.

Comments

Terry's parents were intelligent and well informed. They had no doubts about the honest uncertainty mentioned in note 2. Many a clinical interviewer had been left feeling that he or she had been through an impressively up-to-date viva, and that they hadn't always passed. Paradoxically, what Terry's parents were also looking for was an old-fashioned doctor who would take over full responsibility and tell them what had to be done; except that they knew, intellectually, that their relief wouldn't last, and that such didactic advice was also likely to be arbitrary. In due course they began to deal with this, and to work with the guilt, bitterness and sense of unfocused blame that were among their mixed feelings about their child's handicap and the circumstances surrounding it. Discovering this and learning to handle it was much more difficult than the educational and social learning care plan that eventually helped Terry.

25a Not enough information

Dear Mr and Mrs Watts,

Thank you for your letter about your second thoughts about us contacting Ryan's teachers. Of course we respect your wish for complete confidentiality about him being seen here.[1] However, as we explained when we met, success in managing Ryan's behaviour does depend on the adults who look after him taking a consistent approach with him, and I think it would be a mistake to leave the school out of the picture.[2] Please bear in mind that it isn't our intention to give the school any information about Ryan or yourselves; we would only want to discuss the details of Ryan's behaviour and various ways of handling it, which is already only too well known in the school.[3] If after all you would be willing to let us contact the school, could you let us know before our next appointment?

Yours sincerely, etc.

Notes

1   True, and needs restating.
2   Perhaps obvious in behavioural and developmental terms, but worth affirming.
3   This is also true, but not necessarily understood by patients and families who sometimes assume that professionals gossip with each other about their clientele.

Comments

Leaving aside questions of our clientele's suspicions and the facts of confidentiality, a useful as well as key aspect of consultative technique is that the work done is with what the *consultees* (in this case, Ryan's teachers) want to bring up. This is, by definition, what they know already anyway. Not only is there no need for new information to be given to the school, but to do this would run counter to a basic principle of consultative work, namely for the agenda to be that of the consultees, not the consultant (Steinberg, 1986, 1989, 1993).

There are other situations where parents (or anyone else for that matter) can block discussion or examination of something which is crucial for assessment and management. Parents might want help for a boy or girl threatened with suspension from a school, but without letting the school know he or she is having psychiatric care. This might be just about manageable in some circumstances, but if a significant part of the problem is the relationship between pupil and staff, it may be that there is nothing one can offer without clinic–school contact. It is important that the clinician should be neither over-accommodating nor too rigid about this: what matters is what exchange of information he or she needs to do the job properly. But certainly there can be occasions where work cannot proceed without access to the necessary information, and if so it needs to be made clear; clarifying *why* such contact is needed usually resolves the problem.

25b Too much information

Dear Mrs Matheson,[1]

Thank you for your letter. I am returning the photocopy of the pages from your daughter's diary.[2] I do understand that you are concerned about what you have read. However, I have decided that any risk involved in not using this information is minor compared with the risk of undermining her psychotherapy at this clinic, which has at last got under way.[3] I would, however, urge you and your husband to think about how to bring up your new anxieties at the next family meeting.[4]

Yours sincerely, etc.

Notes

1 Although this is a family or, more precisely, a parental matter (the writer had expressed concern on her husband's part as well as her own) I wanted to, as it were, pass the private material back along as narrow a path as it had come.
2 For rather similar reasons it felt right to refer to 'your daughter' rather than to use her name; bear in mind we are talking about the nuances of a letter like this, not requirements. But I wanted to establish distance from this overture.
3 This was a correct summary of the risks, quite apart from questions of privacy, confidentiality and the maintenance of the boundaries that made work possible.

4 But, while indicating that this route of communication ought to be closed off, I did want to suggest that discussion between the parents about their anxiety and what to do about it should be opened up.

Comments

The photocopies were forwarded with the traditional 'but don't tell her we've showed them to you'. The request to deal with something, but not to let the person concerned know how you know about it, isn't uncommon in adolescent psychiatry. Neither acquiescence nor indignation at the request helps. (The next letter is another example.) The best way to deal with the many problems that come into psychiatry from the periphery, torpedoing the smooth progression of one's neat and tidy treatment plans, is to move the goal posts ('reframe' it, as they say) and to make the altered situation a new focus for work. Thus how the parents are going to handle the anxiety they have about what their daughter wrote, and how they discovered it, is a focus for them. What the clinician or clinical team are going to do about it is another. One can even have as the focus the mystery no one dares talk about for fear of upsetting someone.

But the matter is not necessarily a simple one. Proffered papers might contain suicidal or even homicidal threats ('We told the Doctor, but he didn't want to know'). On the other hand, if we were all preoccupied with the contents of adolescent diaries we could all be in hospital. It is a matter of judging the context – knowing enough at that stage about the patient and the family to balance the risks of one line of action against the risks of another, as was briefly outlined in the letter. But the aim is to find some way of redirecting the request for intervention and the feelings and attitudes it represents into something more consonant with treatment and the ethics of treatment.

26 Something for the teacher

Dear Ms Strachan,

Thank you for your letter about Felicity.[1] I can understand your anxiety, but I can't think of a way of helping her deal with what you describe unless she knows how I've heard about it.[2] May I suggest the following? Why not have another word with her friends, thanking them for their concern,[3] and see if there is any way they could persuade Felicity to see *you*?[4] Perhaps you'd like to phone me to discuss how best to proceed?[5]

Yours sincerely, etc.

Notes

1 An out-patient at a residential school.
2 The task was for me to raise with Felicity her fear that she might be pregnant,

without telling her how I knew. She had confided in two friends who had gone to their teacher for advice, swearing her to secrecy too. I couldn't think of a way to help while keeping everything secret, and it seemed right to say so.

3   Teenagers can be very caring and resourceful with each other, but sometimes apprehensive about involving adults. I expect the teacher would have made a point of thanking the girls (possibly not), but dropping another word of thanks into the mixture at this early stage would, I believed, be an encouragement for the teacher and set the right tone (helpful, and encouraging help), even though I wasn't sure about where we would go from here.

4   Except there was one possible short cut, and an appropriate one: that if the teacher hadn't asked the girls if they could encourage Felicity to come and see her (and from her letter it seemed she hadn't), perhaps she could see if they might do so. It was strange that she hadn't thought to do this, but feelings are infectious, and the feelings here were of a shameful, anxiety-making secret with no way of handling it.

5   There were so many different outcomes and possible implications here that exploring them all would have resulted in a long and muddled letter. What was suggested instead was consultation with the teacher.

Comments

The consultative task, as in the previous case, is to try to gather together the information about the problem, the information about possible solutions, and the power to assist in some way. This applies as much to new matters arising during treatment as at the beginning. The requests in both cases, had they been acceded to, would have had the opposite effect: creating a gap between the information about a problem and the authority to act on it.

This is not the place to discuss all the ramifications of a dilemma like this. The point is that the letter, deliberately brief and friendly, was intended to be a first step in setting up consultation between myself and the teacher and, if possible, between the girls and our patient, to try to track back down the same route (myself to the teacher, the teacher to the girls and the girls to the patient) in the form of being 'anxious to help' rather than anxiety about feeling helpless. However, a line would be drawn at expecting the girls who approached the teacher to do much more. Their task was to check if Felicity would see her teacher after all, which she did, and some joint work with Felicity between the teacher and the clinic became possible, and was useful.

Would a phone call have done as well as a letter? Yes. But the teacher wrote to me, so I wrote back. It seemed to say something about dealing with the episode in the same measured way. It would not have been right to send a fax, for example, quite apart from the lack of privacy.

27 An enquiry about a patient

Dear Mrs Hubbard,

I wanted to acknowledge your letter.[1] I wonder if you could kindly have a private word with the girl you are concerned about,[2,3] and see if she would like you to liaise with her doctor?[4]

Thank you for writing.

Yours sincerely, etc.

Notes

1 Overall, the less said the better here. However, the headteacher's enquiry was well meant and sensitively put, and I thought it important that the letter didn't come across as curt.
2 My letter didn't give the name of the girl about whom the teacher was enquiring. Her letter 'believed' I was seeing Joanna, but even if this was no more than polite phrasing I thought the reply shouldn't include my patient's name.
3 It was probably unnecessary to stress privacy here, but as the situation might have been somewhat anomalous, I mentioned it, fairly lightly, I hope.
4 Here vagueness is all. 'Her doctor' might be myself, her GP or the school doctor (in this case there was this third possibility), and which one would be up to the girl.

Comments

I hope it has been clear from other cases that liaison between clinic and school is usually desirable, if not always essential, and highly valued. This letter is simply to illustrate a different situation, where an older girl in a sixth form college has sought and is using individual treatment without reference to other adults. In general I would be inclined to regard the headteacher, even of a senior girl, as entitled to ask, even though not entitled to a reply without the patient's permission. But how would one respond to an enquiry from, say, a departmental professor, or an employer? It could be none of their business, and the letter accordingly *really* brief.

The next example raises broadly similar issues.

28 Clarifying useful authority

Dear Mr Owen,

Thank you for your letter about Phillip.[1] I think you were right to get in touch, but in the circumstances it would be better to have a word with Phillip and his parents.[2] You could put your expectations to them, and perhaps discuss with them whether they would like to attend here again, or, if they wish, see their family doctor for his suggestions.[3, 4]

Yours sincerely, etc.

Notes

1 The school and the clinic had already been in touch, with permission.
2 However, the new circumstances were such that the decision about what happened next needed to be made independently of the clinic.
3 Another past contact, since abandoned.
4 A copy went to Phillip's family doctor, to forewarn him of the appointment I hoped would be requested.

Comments

The purpose and structure of this letter is again to try to nudge a proposed clinical contact into a more appropriate consultative one. The issue was Phillip's behaviour at school being so bad that suspension was on the cards, not for the first time. The circumstances were that Phillip and his parents were erratic attenders at the clinic, indeed more or less lapsed despite several attempts at re-engaging them. The proposition, from Mr Owen, was that we should try *something* again, because this was the last hope before suspension. With the best of intentions he was asking for one more try, the implication being that the clinic's skill and authority really was needed here. Had Phillip been psychotic this might have been the case, but what was missing wasn't medical authority but the authority of the parents and the school.

Thus, rather than Mr Owen and I joining forces to persuade Phillip back 'for treatment', about which the family were doubtful anyway, it was more appropriate, and more precisely what needed to be conveyed, for the school to explain again its expectations to Phillip if he was to continue there. If the parents then wanted the clinic's help they could approach us with their worry that Phillip might be suspended, with perhaps renewed motivation to make a new treatment contract. Or they could see the school psychologist or their family doctor again. As in the two previous cases, there is an attempt to interrupt the 'short-circuit' (head to clinic) and retrace steps to a more appropriate route, not in the bureaucratic interests of 'normal channels' but so as to engage the most appropriate sources of information, responsibility and authority *en route* (Steinberg, 2000). In the other cases this was in order to preserve confidentiality, or to enable the most appropriate help to be engaged; in Phillip's case this route was necessary to make treatment feasible, and to enable alternative action if treatment was turned down. If his parents still weren't bothered, then seeing the psychologist or psychiatrist might not happen, but at least Phillip would not be left in limbo as someone 'under the clinic' though not attending. Instead, one would hope, he would be identified as *someone's* legitimate concern in the educational system, and, if the matter then became a legal one, Phillip and his parents would have their views represented, and psychological or psychiatric help would still be available if wanted.

29 Anxiety attacks

Dear Mr and Mrs Wallace, Anthony, and Jackie,[1]

As we said at the end of our session today, I am writing to confirm something we agreed we needed to work on. Everyone agrees that you, Jackie,[2] can manage to handle your school work without too much worry or extra hard work. We also agreed there was something of a mystery why you, Anthony, are spending more and more effort and extra time going over work again late at night when everyone else is asleep.[3] Then there is the problem that you feel too wideawake and tense to get to sleep, which spoils the first part of the next day.

One of the things Jackie said when Anthony was having that argument with his mother was that he was very like his father, and you all agreed.[4, 5] Dad[6] then said that he sympathised with your difficulties at school, Anthony, because he'd never been much of a scholar himself, and that was why neither of your parents 'push' you at school. As they say, you were involved with choosing this school, and they've always said that what would make them happy would be for you to be whatever you like, a dustman, a brain surgeon, whatever, and that if you want to leave school at 16 that will be fine, as long as you had some sort of plan for the future.[7] We agreed that it all sounds very reasonable,[8] yet it still leaves you, Anthony, very worried about how you are doing at school, especially with the exams now coming on.

As I said, it may be that we can't find out why you have to work so hard, at least not in time to take a different sort of approach to these exams, so we said that next time we would try to work out some practical ways of helping for the time being.[9] In fact, Anthony, I was worrying a bit myself about whether you were taking all this discussion on your own shoulders as well – how to work very hard at not working too hard![10]

We can talk about this again next time.

Yours sincerely, etc.

Notes

1 The letter was sent to confirm where a session had got to, as agreed.
2 Jackie, Anthony's sister, played an important role, but the rest of the family had been reluctant to bring her to sessions about what was perceived as Anthony's problem. While the observation on Jackie's work was a reminder about her part in the family's feelings about school, it was also to acknowledge the importance of her contribution to the work we were doing in the clinic.
3 I wanted to state this as the main problem – Anthony being up all night – although

the problem had presented as an anxiety state with panic attacks and insomnia, hypochondria about his heart, and fears of dying – i.e. an anxiety-laden disorder which prevented him from working. But it did seem that his feelings about shool work were causing the anxiety.

4 Again, acknowledging Jackie's useful comment.

5 Arguing that was acknowledged as 'to be expected' was that between Anthony and Jackie. The little tussle that broke out between Anthony and his mother was unusual, and embarrassed Anthony and his parents (but not Jackie), and I mentioned this in the letter as something that had been noticed, and was appropriate and useful.

6 I can't justify using 'dad' at this point except to say it felt right. Roles and relationships are kaleidoscopic in such sessions, and sometimes the practitioner is addressing Mr or Mrs Wallace, sometimes referring to 'your father' or 'your mother' and sometimes partially speaking *for* someone, even momentarily, as in 'Do you want to ask mum what she thinks?' Sometimes one uses a parent's first name, even the familiar name the other spouse uses, on that sort of occasion ('Have you asked Mike?'). I mention this not as brilliant strategy, but to make the point that names, too, are words to be used with a little thought and for some therapeutic reason, rather than because one likes to address one's patients in a particular manner.

7 Similarly, my reference here to Anthony's father's story of his school-days and his thoughts about ambition includes the sorts of words and phrases he uses regularly when reassuring Anthony that he doesn't have to be a 'scholar' if he doesn't want to.

8 'Sounds very reasonable' can be a slightly challenging phrase – the wording invites dissent – and I wanted to highlight this for the agenda, especially as the sentence goes on to say that it doesn't seem to work.

9 The exams were looming, the problem seemed rooted in self-perpetuating over-conscientiousness and the family story, and Anthony was going to be trapped in a tighter and more distressing corner. While acknowledging that we were working on long-term and puzzling issues, I wanted to clear a space for short-term strategies and support too.

10 We use the feelings our clients induce in us in different ways, and sometimes should refer to them directly. I also wanted to put something down for my own bit of the agenda for referring to again: that Anthony's over-conscientiousness and anxiety was occuring in relation to the treatment too.

Comments

The formulation I was developing included the power of the unspoken message: that Anthony's father was disappointed in his own school career, and would have loved to see his son 'get on' in ways he never had himself. He was an intelligent, thoughtful man who had built up a successful small business, and the family's life-style was a tribute to this. He also saw – had literally seen among their friends and acquaintances – the results of pushing children too hard academically and imposing frustrated adult ambitions on them – and he and his wife had bent over backwards, indeed made a big thing about their love for the children and their satisfaction in whatever would make them happy, with no particular expectations in terms of educational achievement (an atmosphere in which Jackie was plunging happily ahead, with ambitions, supported by her teachers, to be a vet).

This letter had followed the first session. The following letter was sent after the second.

30 An unexpected finding

Dear Dr Martin,

Further to my earlier letter about Anthony, it emerged in our second session that Anthony has been drinking vast quantities of a cola drink – between two and three litres most nights – while working late on his revision. He finds it helps him to stay awake, and he likes it anyway. He now has a mug of milky tea instead and is feeling a great deal better. He now has no physical symptoms, sleeps well and, although he is still a worrier (particularly about school work and exams), he does not now feel anywhere near as anxious, and is a happier young man all round.

It is interesting that his younger sister Jackie was the first to mention Anthony's nocturnal drinking habits.

I am going to see them again after the exams to review with them what if any further help is needed, and whether the patterns of family relationships mentioned in my earlier letter still need attention.

I have sent a copy of this letter to Anthony and his family.

Yours sincerely, etc.

Comments

I don't think we know what tips the balance in individuals or families and results in a person becoming a patient. I am quite sure that in very many cases it is the accidental and arbitrary nature of the referral process that brings to our attention patterns of behaviour such as that described in Letter 29, yet such patterns of behaviour and variations in personality will be found universally among the families of happy and unhappy, successful and unsuccessful people.

Not that what tips the balance and leads to referral need be taking too much stimulating drink, even in this case. What may impress us intellectually as the components of a compelling formulation may not necessarily carry the same weight for everyone. We might place more weight on a particular aspect (e.g. family or diet) and can always add 'denial' if anyone disagrees. Although we acknowledge the distinction between mechanism and meaning (what happens, but also how much it matters) I think there is a tendency to leap upon the patterns we expect to see and assume they confirm the aetiological picture. We should be sceptical about which causes what in the immense complexity of people's feelings, relationships and behaviour. We should also ask about details of life-style, such as favourite bedtime drinks.

Not that the emerging family formulation became irrelevant the moment the nature of Anthony's nightcap was discovered. Advice about this and about ways of working and revising helped Anthony up to and through the exam, and the fact that the family came together and looked at what school means to them all might have enabled the positive side of the parental message to come through more clearly.

31 Autonomy versus loss of control

Dear Michael,[1]

I'm sorry you decided not to keep our last appointment, but as you know your parents came instead, because they are worried about what to do, and they wanted my advice.[2]

I know things are getting bad[3] for you again, and that you don't want to see us at the moment, although I do remember, quite recently, when you told me that we were helping quite a lot. I think we could help again, and we would like to.[4]

Although I don't know about everything that has annoyed you or disappointed you about our clinic, I do remember that you said you didn't want to talk to me about not seeing your friends, one of them in particular.[5, 7] I remember it because that was one part of our agreement that you didn't want to talk about.[6] Although I was disappointed that you wouldn't agree not to go down to the ——,[8] I thought it was good that you didn't make a promise you weren't going to keep.[9] Anyway, I think that one of the reasons that things have got worse[10] is because you're taking drugs again. I also think that because you've started taking some else's drugs you've stopped taking mine. That's another reason why things have got worse.[11]

I think you ought to come and see me again, and I enclose an appointment card. Please phone if you can't make it.

I've told your parents that I would be writing to you[12]

Yours sincerely, etc.

Notes

1 The letter was to Michael only, but with a copy to his GP. He knew this.
2 Michael's parents had kept an appointment intended for Michael, when he wouldn't attend, and asked me not to tell him. I persuaded them to let me.
3 'Getting bad' was one of Michael's phrases.
4 Perhaps not necessary, but with Michael's particular problems (see Comments, below) I thought the repetition, including affirmation of the wish to help, might be useful.

5 Michael's parents told me how desperately worried they were about him, but while this was reasonable, their constant generalised if understandable anxiety was also part of the problem. I confined myself to one of their specific worries: his friendships.
6 This 'spelling out' and reminiscing is rather clumsy and wouldn't be right for most sorts of letters. Michael's attention and recollection weren't good, and he was sometimes alarmed by people knowing things about him that he wasn't aware he'd told them in the first place. He feared people 'reading his mind', something that was reinforced by an assumption he had that his needs ought to be known by those close to him. He felt quite 'transparent' – his own term – and unsure what was real and what was not. I had found that explaining carefully and step by step what I knew and how I knew it helped sustain reasonably coherent conversations, and I used this style in the letter.
7 A drug-selling 'friend' of Michael whose name I didn't want to state in the letter.
8 'Going down the ——' was Michael's phrase, and one of the few things he managed to do independently, reliably and with a sense of pride and pleasure. I couldn't bring myself to omit the 'to' in my letter; but in any case it would have been too colloquial, too familiar, too much straying into his territory.
9 This comment could perhaps appear a little patronising, or at least paternalistic, but given how Michael was, and what I knew helped his self-esteem, I thought it needed to be said in the context of his also being nagged and admonished.
10 'Things' getting worse rather than 'you' getting worse: euphemistic? Michael had problems distinguishing between feeling bad and 'being' bad, and the colloquialism seemed to me to touch the right note. Again, it was also his way of speaking about his illness. 'I feel bad because I am bad' was one of Laing's particularly precise observations about problems with self-concept (Laing, 1970).
11 There was a clinical responsibility here to spell out how Michael was damaging himself with his self-medication of bought drugs (a variety of soft, admixed and probably bogus substances which included cannabis derivatives, amphetamine and nitrazepam). To these I would add the misuse of alcohol. There was also a wider therapeutic responsibility to try to steer a course between encouraging some aspects of his more independent activities on the one hand and setting limits on the other, which, at his age – an immature 20 – he hated.
12 Michael's ambivalence about his parents was extreme. He simultaneously demanded their support (and subsidies) and furiously resented it. Telling his parents that I would write to him, and also outlining what I was going to say, but without sending them a copy, seemed to me a reasonable balance between his demand for independence and privacy and his dependent behaviour, and something to build into a contract.

Comments

Picking up from notes 10 and 11, these aspects of the letter indicate some of the difficulties of managing a mentally ill adult who is behaving irresponsibly and immaturely but not so acutely self-destructively as to justify compulsory treatment. I would doubt whether his personality and illness would qualify for 'compulsory care in the community' should this dubious hybrid get off the ground in any practical way. Michael was of low average intelligence and, after years of uncertainties about his diagnosis, chronic schizophrenia had been settled for, somewhat reluctantly by psychotherapists who had always sensed that they were nearly helping, but not quite. Several psychotherapies and all the appropriate drugs had been tried. He was just about getting by. In a culture less endowed with clinics, hospitals and hostels, the fact that he was being looked after by his parents, occasionally getting drunk and disturbed in fairly inoffensive and non-threatening ways and heading for chronic dependence, chronic illness and very likely ultimate vagrancy might be regarded as inevitable. His parents had no wish to force him out of their home, and he had no motivation to use a variety of day and group facilities that had been tried. He had refused such offers of residential care that were available. One attempt at a therapeutic community had rapidly fallen through; again, he had not been able to engage in a setting which relied on his motivation. The clientele of places which didn't rely on self-motivation horrified his parents as much as himself.

There is, of course, much more to say about this not uncommon clinical problem of adolescence and young adulthood. Family therapy, including that along the educational lines described by Leff and his colleagues (Leff *et al.*, 1985) had failed through Michael's non-participation, although subsequent work with his parents alone had helped to some extent.

We did our best to 'stand by', as lifeboatmen say, while Michael and his family limped along, helping in what feasible ways we could, and not without hope, and the letter reflects some of this.

Chapter 7

Some special situations

32 What seems to be the trouble?

Dear Mr Johnson,[1]

Thank you for your letter. I find it difficult to know quite how to respond, because we are clearly seeing things in different ways.[2] However, I am of course very sorry that you are so upset.[3] I cannot answer your questions about the young person you asked about, for reasons of confidentiality. With regard to your sister and brother-in-law, I know that they have tried very hard to explain and to reassure you, and my own opinion is that they have now done all they can in this respect, and that if they keep trying fruitlessly, everyone will only get even more upset. I think you are entitled to know that my advice to them is that they may wish to let you know at regular intervals how Howard is doing, but no more than that unless they particularly want to.[4]

I do understand that you feel you are being kept out of the picture, as you say, but I would ask you to appreciate that it is quite difficult maintaining the consistency and predictability that Howard's problems need,[5] even with only his immediate family and ourselves involved, and we cannot accommodate your own interventions and suggestions as well.[6] I must tell you, by the way, that I do disagree with you.[9]

I would like to emphasise that your sister and brother-in-law are both very concerned about how best to respond to you, which is why they asked me to assist.[7,8]

You are quite right, of course, to consider the alternative sources of advice[10] that you mention, and to complain formally if you wish.[11]

Yours sincerely, etc.

Enc.

Notes

1 This letter was marked 'Private and confidential' and sent to Mr Johnson only, with Howard's parents' agreement. (Howard was 12 years old and in a paranoid psychotic state, and for both reasons was not involved in decisions about the correspondence. Had he been older, and less acutely disturbed, he might have been.)

2 This statement has the flavour of 'psychobabble' and euphemism, but what has come to be labelled pejoratively as psychobabble has its purposes and integrity. First, the statement is true. Second, even if it had been wise, kind, honest and sensible to tell Mr Johnson that I thought what he was saying was crazy, it might have been briefly satisfying but would have been less truthful.

3 This was also true, though perhaps the 'very' wasn't necessary.

4 We all know whom we're discussing. Howard's first name is mentioned anyway, and the letter was sent with his parents' consent. However, the somewhat impersonal earlier reference to Howard is a reminder that we (Mr Johnson and ourselves) are by no means all together in a familiar sort of way in this dispute over Howard's care; that there is a boundary here.

5 This is correct, and needed to be said. Mr Johnson might not have known, or thought it was important or to be adhered to.

6 Here and elsewhere we thought it important to emphasise that the clinical team wasn't neutral in a family dispute, but that Howard's parents had our support, particularly since they had tried without success to satisfy Mr Johnson.

7 This too is correct, and appropriately protective. It was easier for the hospital team to distance Mr Johnson than it was for his sister and brother-in-law, a few streets away.

8 Again, an accurate description of the situation, albeit from our perspective. I decided throughout to address Mr Johnson from myself, rather than from 'the team', because he was a dominating man who from the start had demanded the attention of whoever was in charge. We could have made a point by writing back about team decisions, all of us being in agreement, and so on, which might have been right for a dispute with, say, a senior administrator, but not, I think, in this case.

9 Somewhere along the line I thought this statement was needed: that I disagreed with Mr Johnson's demand, which included the intervention of a spiritual healer he knew, and herbal remedies.

10 This was possibly a mistake; I was referring to Mr Johnson's warnings that he was going to contact his Member of Parliament, the High Commission of the family's original country, his solicitor and a number of human rights organisations, but he might have thought I was referring to the medical remedies he was exploring.

11 A copy of the Hospital's Complaints Procedure was enclosed.

Comments

In fact the whole letter might have been something of a mistake. I believe it contains what needs to be said in a situation like this, but it is inclined to the legalistic, and I would place it in the category mentioned on page 21 of letters that make the writer feel better. Even in experienced circles where the dynamics of scapegoating and projection are understood and worked with fastidiously, there are limits, inevitably so, and *someone* is perceived as the baddy, and outside the cosy group of clinical workers and family. One team's bad mother or rogue partner may be another team's patient, indeed possibly once a disturbed child. I mention this not because I think we should have approached Mr Johnson's suggestions more sympathetically, nor even as a reminder of what a tiresomely complicated field psychiatry and family work can be, but because we were treating Mr Johnson like an annoying object rather than a troubled man. A much shorter letter would have been preferable and the above contents brought up instead in a meeting with him. Perhaps it would have made no difference in his case, but it might have in another.

For example:

33 A better letter

Dear Mr Johnson,

Thank you for your letter. I have heard from my colleagues and from Howard's parents that you disagree with our treatment approaches here.[1] As a team we are doing the best we can, with of course your sister's and brother-in-law's full consent, and I think we should continue as we are at present. However, perhaps we should meet to discuss your views[2] and your obvious concern about Howard's well-being.[3] Please call my secretary and we will arrange a mutually convenient time.

Yours sincerely, etc.

Notes

1 The move from the particular (Howard's treatment) to the general (our treatment approaches) is more consistent with a consultative approach, and is one of its distinctions from psychotherapy. In the latter it is commonly useful to bring a general statement down to the particular (for example, from everything is hopeless to the client's sense of hopelessness). In consultative work the *reverse* is usually more helpful (from *this situation's* apparent hopelessness to how a range of cases might or might not be). It also acknowledges the respective authority of myself, my team and Howard's family on the one hand, and Mr Johnson's on the other. We are confirming that we are doing the right thing for Howard in the light of 'our approaches'. Correspondingly, Mr Johnson has a right to his (and his acquaintances') opinions elsewhere. The situation becomes less of a nose-to-nose confrontation, and one actually becomes a little curious about what Mr Johnson's friends might have up their sleeves.
2 At the risk of stating the obvious, this being intrinsic to this book, the writer (as the head man whom Mr Johnson demanded to see) has, in this letter, stepped back to take a wider view of what may conceivably be in Howard's interests, rather than standing in a defensive posture in front of the others.
3 This important observation isn't to be found in the first letter.

Comments (continued)

Howard's family are first generation descendants from immigrants, and Mr Johnson is much more tied to the ways of the 'old country', and much older than his sister, who perceives him as difficult, bossy, intrusive and undermining. There was no question of his involvement in extended family therapy, which would have been the best way of proceeding in some similar circumstances, if only to clarify where authority lay in decisions about Howard's care. He was kept at something of a distance, along the lines outlined in the first letter, and while he remained resentful I believe he felt he was being treated respectfully, and relationships with his sister and brother-in-law were no worse. *En route*, he and his spiritual healing friend came to a meeting with myself and Howard's key workers, accompanied by a senior welfare worker from a human rights group that attended to the affairs of the community concerned. She told us that what Mr Johnson was pressing for bore no relationship whatever to reputable traditional healing in the family's culture, and in fact sounded quite eccentric, if not disturbed.

Although the approach we took was not strictly a consultative exercise, it was closer to consultation than to deploying institutional authority. Elsewhere I have discussed the value of the techniques of consultation in relation to cross-cultural misunderstandings (Steinberg, 1999).

34 To keep trying

Dear Mr and Mrs Carmichael, and Rod,[1]

I enclose a copy of the letter I have sent to your doctor and to the specialist who was seeing Rod. It does suggest a somewhat different approach to what was being tried before, and after our appointment the other day I was left thinking that the degree of difference might lead to some misunderstanding.[2]

Rod's problems are complicated and are now unfortunately long-standing, but I think this is due to the fact that they are difficult to treat, not because the wrong treatment has been tried.[3] Bear in mind that there have been some improvements, especially recently, and that Rod is learning to live with some difficulties, and I don't see why he shouldn't be able to manage better given some more time. He is a brave young man, and although he can get impatient and frustrated I think that is also a good sign of his determination to keep trying.[7]

The disagreement about how to diagnose Rod's illness is not, in my opinion, because we don't know which doctor is 'right', but because we don't yet know enough about this sort of problem or the best way to treat it. There will be some specialists who will speak with more confidence than others about their beliefs and experience, and one of them might have the answer, but from my own experience, that of my colleagues and from what the researchers are saying, I don't believe anybody is in a position to say what is sure to help.[3]

The list of things I have suggested trying in my letter to Doctor Wise will probably make you feel, as you said, that something can be done. I think they are well worth trying. However, unfortunately there is nothing really new there, and it is rather a matter of trying different combinations of treatment and thinking in terms of a sequence for how best to proceed, including repeating some of the tests sometime. It has been easier for me to draw up this list of suggestions because of what has been tried in the past, even if some of it was disappointing. You will see that I am suggesting trying some things again, with more detailed monitoring and 'fine tuning',[4, 9] and persisting for a little longer each time if something helps a little.[5] In fact I think the only two new things I am suggesting are, first, looking again at what helped a little before, even if it was ultimately disappointing, and, second, building in definite times when key people on the team can review progress with you.[5, 8]

I think a painstaking review of progress with whoever is helping would be well worthwhile, say once or twice a year, but you may like to think of asking for more regular meetings to discuss both progress and disappointments.[5] You could also think over whether some meetings just for yourselves, as parents, without Rod, might help.[6]

So that everyone knows what is being said,[8] I have sent a copy of this letter to the others. Perhaps you could discuss it with Dr Wise?[10]

Yours sincerely, etc.

Notes

1 This was a somewhat difficult letter to write for reasons discussed in the Comments (below). That is probably why it is too long. I addressed it to Rod (who was 18 years old and had a personality disorder which had been described as autistic spectrum, obsessional and schizotypal), and his parents, rather than the whole family (an older and a younger sibling), because it was Rod's and his parents' choice that only the three of them came to the appointment.

2 I did want to draw attention to a real difference in management, yet as the letter goes on to show, the difference is more one of form than content.

3 But while I wanted to acknowledge a suggested change of approach, I was concerned about the way in which my advice was being taken. The family left giving many thanks and with a sense of euphoria which had complex origins, and, I thought, included an implicit invitation to join in with criticism of present and previous psychiatrists, psychologists and paediatricians who had at various times tried to help. I did think this was a misunderstanding, and had I not felt that a more sober letter would correct the balance, and touch on the sadness of the situation, I would have suggested another appointment to talk over my advice. But see note 6.

4 I think this tends not to happen. I am indicating a difference between that which is intrinsically hard to do if not idealistic (for example, to find a drug which will provide the 'magic' cure), and that which is *not* so very hard to conceptualise and do, but *is* hard to organise and sustain (for example, long-term help from senior, experienced workers in two or three appropriate areas (for example, family

therapy and behavioural psychology) with trials of well-established forms of management and detailed monitoring). Why is this so hard to put in place? At least it can be recommended to parents in a letter, even if it seems like pie in the sky.

5 I have attempted to distinguish here, as elsewhere in the book, between a disease process (characteristically the province of experts, intangible and feared) and the resulting problems and disabilities, which are amenable to common-sense handling, accessible, and perhaps saddening rather than panic-inducing. Anxiety may be the better emergency reaction, but sadness, within reason, is potentially more creative (e.g. Skynner, 1975).

6 Hence the idea being suggested that regular work on family and parental feelings might have a place too.

7 I think it is important to say something positive alongside a message which necessarily contains negatives, providing it is true.

8 For all that isn't possible there is much that is, but it filters through slowly, and the exigencies of staff training and professional progress mean that at any given time a clinical team is fortunate if it has the right people on hand to put in place the treatment for which the best evidence is available *and* see it through for long enough *and* deal with the feelings specifically associated with chronic disorder and disability. There is real progress in broad swathes of psychiatric practice, but the dynamics and politics of teams, departments and career structures tend to be antithetical to putting what is possible into practice. One cannot put all this in a letter, nor should one propose utopian solutions, but if there seems to be a common-sense way forward I think patients and relatives are entitled to know one's views about it.

9 In the end the suggestions are seriously meant to help, but they are undramatic: to see what has helped most, to try it again, and keep trying while reviewing progress. 'Fine tuning' was a metaphor that seemed to carry meaning when we discussed things with Rod and his parents. The essence of the message was to not lose sight of progress, even though there was no cure, and to continue to *expect* long-term collaboration with the available experts; perhaps even giving them some encouragement and ideas.

10 As specialists accumulate around a long-standing, difficult problem, the weight distribution can end up meaning that no one is actually responsible for anything very much. Countries with a general practitioner system, and families that use them, are able to step back from highly complex networks of professional involvement of varying and overlapping aims and characteristics, and, with the help of a highly trained generalist, review where they have got to and what action is needed next. I really wasn't sure which of the quite large group of psychiatrists, psychologists, psychotherapists, specialist teachers and therapists, social workers and others who had been involved with Rod over the past fourteen years would continue with the case (the most recent psychiatrist was not expecting to continue), and I thought that discussing the next step with the family doctor held out the best chance for some continuity.

Comments

This case has similarities with Letter 24, and in fact such situations are common, particularly as older adolescents with chronic problems enter young adulthood. Whatever remedial clinical techniques are available (or ever will be), the essential nature of the problem is likely to be developmental; that is to say, complexly interacting variations from the norm developing as the individual grows, rather than a circumscribed disease process. This means in turn that the help needed is likely to require a fairly extended period of education, rehabilitation, the systematic shaping up of skills, and work that helps sustain the individual and family in their normal life, and to maintain treatment with energy and the right balance of optimism and realism. This is not easy, but it is feasible and practical and the skills are there, for example, in teaching, psychological, psychotherapeutic and social work professions. What tends to be missing are workers who stay long enough in one place to form a viable interdisciplinary team, gain experience from it and stay with patient and family for long enough, and who are able to take a necessarily experimental approach, each patient acting, so to speak, as his or her own control. These very different styles of work can be found together in child and adolescent psychiatry (Steinberg, 1983, 1986, 1987), where in my view they provide a sound model for all psychiatric care, but not so often in the adult field (Tyrer and Steinberg, 1998). But even children's psychiatric, psychological and care services generally can fall short, providing a first-rate service for a small number who 'get through' but leaving large gaps, as much because of the way a multiplicity of services is organised and the rather rigid way we sometimes think in these fields, as because of 'inadequate resources'. When some time ago I made such points in a book (Steinberg, 1981), they seemed to cause a number of academic reviewers of the time some pain, though, interestingly, the book's argument has remained popular with front-line practitioners.

To return to the letter. I was trying to say that something special is needed, but it was in the realms of common sense (persistence, trying things out, sticking with it, monitoring progress, working on small gains) rather than a scientific 'breakthrough'; but common sense augmented by the sort of observational, treatment planning and fine-tuning skills our professions ought to have: applied attention to detail. It also requires that empathy and open-mindedness that tells us when to stand back, when to simply support and encourage and when to think in terms of individual and family psychodynamics, which I hope was implicit in the letter.

With the sorts of long-term conditions that are always going to be with us, the best we can do is exchange impossible expectations for ones that are merely extremely difficult to put in place. I have no doubt that there are sound if not sane psychological reasons why we organise things how we do. Are career structures designed to maintain a distance from large numbers of long-term, difficult problems? Perhaps with imagination we can find other ways to keep professional spirits up and work on track.

35 Informing the family doctor

Dear Mr and Mrs Smith,

Thank you for your fax and messages. I felt I should explain further my message to you via my secretary.

I'm sorry if my request – that your son's[1] family doctor should know of and approve my seeing him – causes any difficulties. I am in full agreement that confidentiality is extremely important.[2] However, I do think it essential that a general practitioner should know if a specialist is seeing one of his or her patients. I believe this would be in your son's interests, for advice about which specialists to see, and as a focus for the advice given, past, present and in the future. If one doctor isn't aware of what another is doing, or even what is thought about a case, there is a risk of conflicting advice and incompatible treatment. Even if there were no such dangers in your son's case, I think something is being lost if he doesn't have the benefit of the two perspectives, one general and the other specialised.[3]

You need to know that not all consultants would agree with me on this point. My secretary has given you the names of two others in my field in the —— area. I don't know their views, and hope that they will be able to help.[4]

Let me know, however, if this presents insuperable problems.[5]

With kind regards.

Yours sincerely, etc.

Notes

1   I thought it was better to refer to 'your son' rather than to use his name. I would have felt I was being slightly overfamiliar talking about Nick by name without knowing if he was aware of the referral, and without having any plans to see him. Not the most important of points, but worth a second's thought. It also maintains a little distance in a situation in which, I sensed, roles and boundaries might not be clear.
2   This is quite enough. I initially added something about how highly confidentiality ranked in my priorities, but decided it was not only unnecessary but rather prim as well.
3   Mr and Mrs Smith were entitled to an outline of my reasons, though an extended argument (see Comments, below) would have been inappropriate. I was going to remind them that this was in their son's interests, i.e. it wasn't merely a bureaucratic position, but that should be clear from the reasons, and didn't need rubbing in as if I were more concerned about their son than they were.
4   It was important to point this out. I don't believe I'm alone on this subject, but if on balance the wording seemed to suggest that I was the eccentric here, rather than whichever consultant agreed to see them, that was alright.
5   I thought this was also important. One cannot know all the circumstances behind a

case. My secretary had gathered that they did have a family doctor, although they wouldn't say why they did not want him to know about the referral. In addition, while the matter was apparently pressing, it wasn't an emergency: they had been happy with an appointment initially offered two or three weeks hence in return for their doctor's referral. It was a private referral, so I wasn't their only option, as can now be the case in many sectorised services. For these reasons I thought it logical that they should approach someone else, but special reasons can justify unusual procedures, and I didn't want to close the door, at least not to further consultation about the matter.

Comments

Letter 35 was an example of a case where, it seemed to me, the family doctor's role is an important one to preserve. I don't know how many would agree with me, but in any case my purpose here is to demonstrate a way of putting a particular view in a letter, not promoting it.

36 An awkward question

Dear Jane,

Thank you for your letter. I don't know what to make of your first session with the therapist either.[1] I would say, though, that the approach which most psychotherapy takes is a little away from the ordinary, because it tries to help with problems for which ordinary conversations (including conversations with oneself) haven't been enough.[2] However, Dr Z—— will be interested in what you think, so why not talk to her about what you told me and see what happens?[3]

I hope you find it worth persisting with.[4] Let me know sometime how you get on.[5]

Yours sincerely, etc.

Notes

1 I could have written 'from your account' but that would have been a little condescending or legalistic, or both. She would know I was referring to her account, and there was no need to affirm it. However it is worth framing the second sentence in this sort of letter in a way that will jog one's memory if looked at years later, rather than writing an extended introduction or heading.
2 I thought this attempt at a one-sentence explanation of psychotherapy might help.
3 This was rather close to the boundary, because I don't think one should tell someone how to use their psychotherapy session. However, I don't believe it went over it.
4 As well as being genuinely meant, and leaning on the side of optimism, this is also a reminder that continuing in psychotherapy is in the client's hands.

5 I spent more time wondering about saying this than composing the rest of the letter. It is a touch protective, and others might not have included this invitation. My intention was to show interest without distracting from her source of care.

Comments

Jane was an ex-patient of a few years back who had been referred by her family doctor to Dr Z—— for psychotherapy. This had been part of the longer-term plans with which I had discharged her (see Letter 39). I knew only a little about the psychotherapist. As is occasionally the case (with psychiatrists too) she was a slightly controversial, individualistic figure, and although there were no doubts about her professional experience and integrity, some people (mostly rather mainstream psychiatrists and psychologists) thought her style a touch eccentric. I had met her once briefly at a conference and found her pleasantly unexceptional and commonsensical.

So there you are. When I refer someone for psychotherapy I anticipate the first session to be one of mutual sizing up. This is almost always the therapist's policy anyway. I wasn't so sure here, and had suggested the referral some time previously, rather than making it myself. The patient was also still quite young. So I expressed the curiosity I actually felt, though if she had come back with serious doubts my advice would have been that she discuss these doubts with the referring GP.

What she had written about was the psychotherapist's apparent vagueness and long silences, and felt she wasn't being helped to talk and didn't know what to tell her. She also said they both gazed out of the window quite a lot.

Should I assume that all readers of this book will know the ways of psychotherapists? There are more styles of psychotherapy than there are drugs in the British National Formulary. Some are active and directive at the cognitive and behavioural end of the spectrum, while at the psychoanalytical end I believe a session could consist of fifty minutes' silence if the patient doesn't say anything. Brown and Pedder (1979) provide an excellent review. Different people and different problems need very different approaches, and there is a place and a rationale on this very broad spectrum for the therapeutic strategy where the therapist determinedly expects the patient to take the initiative, on the principle that what surfaces (characteristically along the lines 'I thought you'd tell me what to do') is a good place to start. However, it takes wisdom on both sides to make it work and if appropriate persistence.

37 Someone has to pay

Dear Mr Berk,

My secretary tells me that your account has not been settled,[1] despite her sending a second reminder last month. Of course I can't know the reason for this,[2] and I don't know whether there's a practical problem or whether it's something that we ought to discuss in one of our sessions.[3] Could you let me know?[4]

Yours sincerely, etc.

Notes

1 The statement of fact is important, whatever the tone of the letter. After all, the recipient might not know.
2 Non-payment of an expected sum of money is one of the great feeling and fantasy generators on both sides. It is worth acknowledging that at this point neither participant yet knows what is in the other's mind about this transaction. Thus –
3 all possibilities can be allowed for. The payments might be accumulating in someone's in-tray. The patient might be angry with the clinician, or disappointed and holding on to the payment as a sort of hostage. Some workers hope for payment by return of post, others within a few months. If the clinical work is psychotherapy, the reason might be a useful focus for a time.
4 This leaves the ball properly in the other's court.

Comments

Correspondence about bills could make an interesting book. I wanted to mention it here simply to identify a taboo. It is astonishing how workers who can comfortably discuss sex, death and worse can become quite apprehensive, tongue-tied and even angry about money, especially, of course, if income happens to be laundered tidily through state agencies, grant awarding bodies and so on.

38 The best policy

Dear Mr and Mrs West, Peter and Sally-Ann,

I enclose a copy of the report sent as requested to your insurance company.[1] You will see that I have described your problem, Peter, under the heading mental disorder, and added a code that is used in classifying psychiatric conditions. This is the sort of thing the insurance company wants to know.[2]

Although in the family meetings we have agreed that Peter's angry and upset reaction to what happened was pretty much normal and understandable, and not the psychiatric illness people thought at first it might be, the fact is that for administrative reasons (e.g. for your insurance policy) it does come under that sort of heading. I don't believe I am misleading you, Peter, or the insurance company, if we describe what has happened in these two sorts of ways, although it is rather confusing.[3]

We can talk about this if you wish next time.[4]

Yours sincerely, etc.

Notes

1 Having provided a report with, necessarily, Peter's and his family's permission, I assume they will read it.
2 They might not have noticed or bothered about the terminology referred to. I thought there was no harm done and perhaps some advantage if they did.
3 I thought this was worth saying.
4 This too.

Comments

The issue is an important practical one (i.e. Peter and his family's perception of what happened, the implications for treatment, and their entitlement to use their insurance cover for psychiatric illness) but also a philosophical conundrum.

Bolton and Hill (1996) have discussed the definition of psychiatric disorder as well as can be found anywhere, and much hinges on the issue of the causes of a state of mind and its understandability. If Peter's misbehaviour had been shown to be due to a brain tumour, or if a genetically loaded change in his neurochemistry could be demonstrated, then one criterion of illness would be met. However, there was no reason to think that he (or his family) understood his quite damaging anger and distress until it emerged that he had been far more upset by the death of a friend whose family his own family disliked than had been suspected. On the contrary, he had said, and believed, that it wasn't important. His containment of one set of feelings about the death, and his subsequent explosiveness when his parents crossed him in various fairly ordinary ways, had complicated roots to do with his loss, his adolescence, and the way his family tended to handle feelings and conflict. Peter (and his parents) had no more reason to be familiar with thinking of causation along such lines than with neuroanatomy or biochemistry. Yet the treatment, a combination of individual counselling, behavioural guidance and family work, involved Peter and his family learning new perspectives on what had happened and sharing responsibility for putting it right. This required quite a substantial change of position from 'Peter as ill' to 'Peter as furious about something we now understand', and a shift from 'Please do something about it' to 'Help us do something about it'.

I would not have gone on about it at such length if such considerations didn't apply to great swathes of psychiatric disorder (or conditions, or illness). The implications go well beyond the pragmatic, operational needs of insurance companies, and like pragmatic, operational needs they make us think. So *did* Peter have a mental illness? The accurate and truthful answer is: yes and no.

Chapter 8

Endings

39 Looking Ahead

Dear Dr Carson,[1]

As mentioned in my last letter, I have now discharged Jane —— from my clinic, having had a final session with her and her parents the other day. Her diet and weight have remained normal for some months and her menstrual cycle is returning to a regular pattern. She is cheerful and confident, has rebuilt her social life, and her school reports are fine, and she is expected to gain university entrance next year. There is no trace now of a weight phobia, and her bafflement[2] at how she once allowed her weight to fall so dramatically without apparent concern is characteristic of someone who has been through a period of severely disturbed thinking.

She now wants no further contact with the psychiatric clinic and wishes to get back to her studies and her normal life. I have every sympathy with her wishing to put all this behind her, and if there is a little denial and a lot of optimism operating then that can also be part of the recovery process.[3]

I think, on balance, that she will be fine, but I have asked Jane to make an appointment to see you in three months to check that her weight and menstrual cycle are alright, partly to keep a non-psychiatric eye on her but also so that her mother will not feel she has to keep checking on how she is doing.[4] However, I do think Jane would[5] benefit from individual psychotherapy focused on her self-esteem and self-worth, even if she is unwilling and perhaps unable to make full use of it now. I suggested she waits until she feels there has been a gap that feels long enough, by which time she will I think[6] have moved away from home and be settling in another part of the country, and to then reconsider psychotherapy,[7] approaching her current general practitioner about this in the first instance.[8]

I have discussed the contents of this letter fully with Jane and her parents at our last session, and have sent Jane a copy.[9]

Yours sincerely, etc.

Notes

1 This is an example where I thought a doctor-to-doctor letter, read by Jane, might be more likely to receive attention and be remembered than a letter written directly to her.

2 There was cheerful astonishment at the near-delusional state of unconcern she had been in, as her weight fell relentlessly and her body chemistry became increasingly disturbed, which can be seen in young people making an excellent recovery as well as in those who still have some psychological work to do. In the last two sessions we had acknowledged both possibilities, though Jane was amused at my caution. She likened it to the anxious intrusiveness on her mother's part which had been a focus for family therapy, and which we had acknowledged to have been appropriate and necessary at one stage. I thought the word 'bafflement' was about right; it is a 'light' enough term but nevertheless indicates something not understood.

3 I think this is true and needed to be said. The term 'denial' was familiar to her.

4 The proof of the pudding, however, was going to be in these important physical criteria, and seeing her GP seemed entirely appropriate as well as making a contribution to taking weight-preoccupation out of the household.

5 It was interesting that I nearly wrote 'could', a neatly bureaucratic cop-out word. *Would* was what I meant.

6 'I think' is sometimes useful padding in an intense sentence, like 'perhaps'; or something soothing to maintain the reader's tolerance of a rather bossy message. However, I meant it here; negotiating independence (in practice, choosing a university either away from home or within commuting distance) was coming up as rather a crucial decision that had yet to be made.

7 I thought she was right not to want to begin psychotherapy now; and I certainly felt it was psychotherapy that she needed, not counselling (see Comments, below).

8 This too indicated the truly fresh start which seeking psychotherapy was supposed to be. As mentioned elsewhere, I do not think one should be paradoxical in a letter, or at least no more than one can help. However, there is a paradox here in the real situation, and a useful one, in that by really ending treatment, i.e. being properly discharged from *psychiatric* care (with even medical supervision being non-psychiatric) I thought there was a possibility of psychotherapy being sought one day by Jane as an autonomous choice.

9 This is important. The letter was one which affirmed the discussion and planning that had come out of a family session and an individual one. I don't think it would be right for such thoughts and suggestions, least of all from specialist to referrer, to have come up *de novo* in this way.

Comments

This letter alluded to the pros and cons of psychotherapy, but also to its nature, and how it is entered into. If Jane had a pivotal problem amidst all the complexities, it was to do with her sense of autonomy. Paradoxically, to use the psychotherapeutic help I thought she needed, it would be best if she made her own decision about it. On the other hand she was quite young, and work with adolescents is full of ambiguities which don't arise with older people and children.

We could have recommended counselling; I have often, of course with the patient's agreement, put young people in touch with campus counselling services or their equivalent when they've gone on to further training and education, or at least checked (for example, through the prospectus) that there is one available. In Jane's case I think it would have fudged the issue. There was, we concluded, a major difference between 'looking after' Jane when she was at significant risk, and which was initiated and indeed insisted upon by her parents and the professionals they had called in, and the psychotherapy that would help her find other ways of handling stress and conflict. Hence the importance of the 'gap' and the fresh start. The former was a child's position, the latter that of an adult. With counselling, there was the risk of it being perceived as something in between, straddling a gap that would be better left. Whatever the merits of the decision to proceed this way, the point is that the letter was intended to reflect it.

The similarities and differences between psychotherapy and counselling are almost ineffable. I'm sure many readers will know of clear-cut definitions that differentiate them, but there is a wide middle ground in which one can regularly find people who call themselves counsellors practising psychotherapy and people who call themselves psychotherapists practising counselling. There is a case for calling all treatment through conversation in words or symbols psychotherapy (it means of course treatment *by* the mind, not *of* the mind) and differentiating between different levels of intervention, for example, behavioural psychotherapy, cognitive psychotherapy and dynamic psychotherapy. I would say, perhaps simplistically, that in counselling the emphasis is on the counsellor's and the client's conscious thinking about the self or daily life or plans, and may stay that way throughout; while the emphasis of dynamic psychotherapy is on the unconscious processes that influence these things. Probably, however, an intensive three-day conference on the subject might well still end in disagreement.

40 Not making it

Dear Mr and Mrs Grant, Denny, Liza and Adam,

Thank you for the further message. I do understand that it's become difficult[1] to get everyone together for the appointments, but it seems to me that the inconvenience all round, plus all of us being quite busy trying to meet when no treatment is really under way, could actually be worse than no treatment at all.[2] By this I mean that it could make us feel that something was being done when it isn't. After thinking carefully about what's best for the children I don't think I should offer another appointment, but suggest that you have another word with your family doctor and with Denny's and Liza's headteachers and make a new start on getting some help.[3] I do think you should do this.[4]

Could you show this letter to the children too? Thank you.[5]

Best wishes. I hope things go better next time.[6]

Yours sincerely, etc.

cc. Dr Barkworth
    The school heads

Notes

1   This is somewhat polite and euphemistic: the truth if not the whole truth, which
    was about the chaos in this family and the doubtful motivation, about treatment, on
    the part of the parents. The children (and all five of them, in a way) were aware of
    this to varying degrees, and it was important that they knew this was why attempts
    at treatment were being stopped, and not for fantasised reasons. I thought it was
    sufficient to say no more than that it had proved too difficult to meet: first, because
    the other reasons would need to be part of sustained therapy, if ever, and second,
    because Mr and Mrs Grant were doing the best they could thus far, and the children
    should see them being treated with respect, and as adults, and not castigated, as can
    happen.
2   This is incontrovertible. While a degree of negotiation and compromise is bound to
    be part of the psychiatrist–patient relationship, the impression that something is
    being done when nothing much is being done can be not only counter-therapeutic
    but in some circumstances dangerous.
3   For similar reasons, those who initiated the referral needed to know what wasn't
    happening, as well as, one hopes, helping to make alternative plans. I didn't
    specifically ask Mr and Mrs Grant for permission to give the heads a copy of this
    letter, but this was because I had already liaised, with permission, with the two
    schools concerned. However, as already said, one must be cautious about confiden-
    tiality, and a similar letter about similar circumstances could be open to allegations
    that one was saying rude things about Mr and Mrs Grant's capacity as parents. What
    to say to whom depends of course on the degree of risk to the child, but one can get
    permission more often than not, and it is always possible to put things kindly.
4   I wrote this in case it wasn't clear.
5   I guessed that both Mr and Mrs Grant would read the letter, but I doubted
    whether the children would see it. I added this in the hope that it would make it
    slightly more likely. There are occasions when children become more interested in
    therapy than their parents, and it would then be important to write directly to them.
    Of course there are also circumstances where children need to continue to be seen,
    regardless of the parents' involvement, and we can then be in complex areas of
    childcare where the parents' attitudes and behaviour could be questioned, and other
    authority sought to enable treatment to continue. This is not the place or the book
    to discuss this; suffice it to say that the letter illustrates just one aspect of this
    important and potentially difficult area. However,
6   this wasn't the heaviest or gloomiest of cases; other options were feasible for the
    schools and the family doctor, and, just as important, I believed something useful
    would be learned from the message of the letter. I did know from the history of
    previous treatment that it would have come as a surprise. Hence ending on a
    friendly and positive note felt right.

Comments

This letter was about non-attendance, characteristically following phone calls and letters that apologised profusely and made extravagant promises about next time. A broadly equivalent letter could have been written about families which dutifully attend but are unable and unwilling (the two being reciprocal to an extent) to put into practice what the therapy needs – for example, a particular behavioural strategy. This can become a new focus for therapy but will not necessarily work. Unless children are at risk, or are themselves wanting help, it can be appropriate to arrange a pause, as in this case.

41 Saying thank you

Dear Judy,

It was very kind of you to write the way you did. It cannot have been easy to do so, and it doesn't surprise me at all that there's been such a long gap before you felt able to write. I do remember the very difficult sessions, and you certainly did make your feelings very clear. You did indeed once break the door. For a long time we seemed always to be starting again, but more recently something more positive seemed to have begun and that seemed to be the time when you appeared to feel less angry too about other things in your life, present and past. I think it was good when you made it by yourself to the job centre and that you got through some interviews that seemed very difficult. It sounds like there were one or two where it was good that you managed to stick with it, instead of walking out, as you once might have done.

I'm glad things are settling down now between yourself and John, and the flat sounds nice. It's good to hear that you are on better terms with your mother too.

Thank you again for writing. It was good to hear from you. Let me know how you get on.

My very best wishes for the future.

Yours sincerely, etc.

Comment

In fact this letter went on and on in much the same vein for several paragraphs more before juddering to an end. Would an ex-patient really welcome a letter like that? Would he or she read it? It seems to convey work undone, ends untied, a need to reminisce about good times and bad, repair work on paper. There's also something spooky about repeating what the patient has said. Why do we do this? Is it because we suspect the writer might have forgotten what they wrote by the time they get our reply? Or perhaps to demonstrate that we read it, line by line? Or is it because we see opportunities in parts of the patient's letter for just a little more therapy, advice or wisdom?

Letters from patients that acknowledge the end – they can be quite long – is an occasion for them, not you, to reminisce and tell anecdotes. They are written to check that you're still there (and that they were), and to say thanks. There's no need to reciprocate in full and line by line, although you should answer questions.

I don't think you should invite further correspondence unless there's a good reason, for example, when after a long period of therapy or admission a vulnerable ex-patient has the task of settling down in a new life, perhaps in a hostel or residential home. Writing can then help them to gently disengage from the care of yourself and your colleagues and begin to engage with new helpers and friends. Of course this initially somewhat lonely and precarious life might be taking place 'in the community', not in an institution. But that sort of letter is a form of continuing therapy, rather than an ending.

A better letter to send would be as follows.

42 Ending

Dear Judy,

Thank you for your letter, and your very kind remarks. It was nice to hear from you. I'm glad everything sounds so much more settled at last.

My very best wishes for the future.

Yours sincerely, etc.

Chapter 9

What recipients think of letters

People in the psychiatric, psychotherapeutic and similar fields with whom I have discussed writing to patients about their conditions and treatment have without exception agreed with me that it is a good thing. Since I am thinking of questions and discussion at the end of lectures as well as informal conversations in the corridor, my 'sample' of professional opinion probably amounts to about two hundred people. In a paper on the therapeutic use of narrative as applied in letters, however, Goldberg (1996) mentioned ways in which letters could be counterproductive and presumably unpopular with some recipients, along the lines discussed in Chapter 2, but also because, if they are not received, whether actually or metaphorically, as intended when they were sent, misunderstanding and miscommunication can be compounded. Privacy may be compromised, again actually or in terms of subjective feeling. I think the latter is quite important; if, as those of us exploring written communication suggest, the letter really is in effect a transitional object conveying and containing something significant about therapy, what might it subtract from the therapeutic session itself as a special, private place and occasion? Might the letter diminish this?

The question therefore arises: what do the recipients of such letters think? A number of papers have raised questions about the value of some letters for some groups of clientele. Thomas (1998), for example, found that letters sent to patients about their condition seemed least welcomed by those with lower levels of educational attainment and those diagnosed as having schizophrenic illnesses. He observed that the very groups for whom engagement in dialogue about the nature of their problems (for example, through the process of writing letters) was most needed seemed least likely to want to engage in it. He also suggested that it was paternalistic to assume that patients were bound to like receiving such letters, even though policies such as opening up notes and letters to patients are generally assumed to be part of a move away from medical paternalism.

In a study of psychiatric out-patients' reactions to letters summarising their consultations, Asch et al. (1991) found that most people reacted positively, seventeen out of twenty-three recipients being pleased to receive them, nineteen finding them easy to understand, and twenty-one very or 'quite' accurate, but only eleven found the letters very helpful, and a further six 'quite helpful'. Three people found the letters upsetting, the reasons given being related to the facing of reality prompted by the letter and by concern about confidentiality. In this admittedly small group, confidentiality did seem to be a general rather than a specific concern (for example, about other members of the household seeing it) because in this study most respondents chose to show the letter to someone else. However, it did raise for me the possibility that seeing private problems set out on paper, even in a confidential letter, might for some people detract from the private intimacy of the treatment relationship, being one of the ways in which it might be perceived as diminished. It could also be a reminder and possibly a source of anxiety about what else is on file, and who else might see it.

Gauthier (1999) reviewed the practice of writing letters to families in the light of the successive legislation in recent years which increases patients' rights of access to their medical records, showing the many ways in which such openness complements and assists therapy, and also making the point that perhaps a distinction ought to be recognised between a clinician's notes about patients and his or her private thoughts, feelings, hypotheses and impressions about them.

Pierides (1999) has pointed out how little data there are on psychiatric patients' reactions to receiving letters about their conditions and treatment, though this has been done in the fields of gastroenterology (Eaden *et al.*, 1988) and general practice (Albert, 1991) with high levels of favourable response. However, he also makes the important point that in cognitive analytic therapy (e.g. Ryle, 1982) writing to patients about the initial formulation and its implications, about 'homework' guidelines and planned areas of work and a 'goodbye' letter on discharge is routine.

A survey of recipients' views: response of patients and families

The above studies show that systematic research into the usefulness of letters would have to take account of the purpose, form and content of letters and the characteristics of the people responding to them as well as to the specific questions being asked. In the short survey that follows, we thought we would simply try to gauge the general feelings of recipients about receiving such letters, as a first and relatively superficial attempt to tap into reactions.

The letters used were in the category of detailed clinical letters about out-patient referrals to the referring general practitioner, with a copy of the same letter to the adolescent patient and his or her family. (They were not, as is explained at the beginning of the Preface, letters that appear in this book.) Short questionnaires were sent out during a two-month period to the last twenty-two patients and families seen for a full clinical assessment (as an ordinary referral or for a 'second opinion') up to the beginning of that period. The letters enquired about in the questionnaires had mostly been sent out in the previous few months, though with one (three-year) exception the other 'long-term' letters had been to patients and families still attending the clinic. The clinic was in the independent sector, and, though the patients were about evenly divided between those who were self-financing (mostly insured) and those who were referred under the Health Service extra-contractual referral system, all would have been categorised as in the middle to upper economic groups, and their educational level would have been equivalent to those whom Thomas (1998) found to be generally positive about such letters. (This was in contrast to young people referred as secondary or tertiary referrals and who had been admitted, the majority of whom were funded by departments of social services or by their health authorities, and whose socio-economic and educational levels were weighted more towards the educational groups which Thomas had found to be less positive.)

The questionnaires were deliberately made very brief, asking only if the original letter was recalled, whether it was remembered as 'very', 'slightly' or 'not at all' helpful, and with space for comments. They were accompanied by stamped addressed envelopes for return.

Twelve questionnaires out of twenty-two sent to patients and their families were returned, all apparently completed by parents. They all reported being pleased to receive the original letter, and all found them very helpful, except for one who found it only 'slightly' helpful, attributing this to it being only a single appointment.

The reasons given for the letters being helpful included the information they contained, for example, about the referred patient and proposals for treatment and care, one respondent seeing the letter as potentially helpful for future reference. The letters were also seen to be clarifying, comforting, supportive, providing a starting point for the next meeting, and offering a 'personal touch'. Although none reported the letters to be unhelpful, one parent reported the patient as being too depressed and negative about paperwork to show interest in the letter, and one reported dissatisfaction that advice given in the letter had not been implemented.

Response of referring doctors

Eighteen out of twenty-two questionnaires sent to referrers (all GPs) were returned. These questionnaires too were extremely brief, and asked the doctor whether it was important that his or her opinion should be sought for sending patients copies of clinical letters, about whether such letters *in general* were likely to be helpful or not, and whether the particular letter in question had or hadn't been helpful.

Most doctors (two-thirds) didn't recall being asked if they agreed to copies of their letters being sent to the patients (all had been), and just over two-thirds didn't think this was important anyway, except (two respondents) if sensitive information from the GP would have been disclosed.

Fifteen of the eighteen family doctors thought that letters like this *in general* were likely to be helpful; the reasons given were particularly interesting and all are listed: that it is helpful to be open with the patient and this encourages trust; that it keeps the patient informed of the consultant's intentions and provides a chance to 're-digest' information, and that keeping patients well informed is particularly important in psychiatric care; that there should be no secrets in clinical medicine; that information and insight (into family dynamics too) helps, including aiding recovery; that clarifying problems reduces anxiety, confusion and suspicion; that it clarifies management strategies, and involves patients and doctors in care plans, in particular helping with discussion of difficult areas.

Such areas of doubt expressed about such letters *in general* were entirely to do with being cautious – that there could be circumstances and occasions when letters like these might be unhelpful, although hypothetical examples weren't given.

Ten doctors thought the letters were helpful in their particular patient's and family's case, very much along the lines given above, with additional comments such as that the letter provided a 'quality check', that it gave a 'clear, detached outline of action', and that it acknowledged areas of disagreement.

Eight doctors didn't know whether or not the letter had been helpful, largely because of lack of or loss of contact with the patient and family or because the letter wasn't recollected. None reported the letter as unhelpful.

Some conclusions

The sample was extremely small and this severely limits the conclusions that can be drawn. Overall, response to the letters was positive, particularly from the family doctors. The response was very positive from those of the client group who returned their questionnaires, but only just over half did so. Those who didn't may have included some, or many, who had not found the letter helpful.

We had invited a confidential response in the hope of encouraging the free expression of views. Unfortunately, this meant that we were not able to match response with diagnosis or educational attainment, both of which Thomas' study (1998) had shown to be significant in some respects, but on the other hand the latter seemed to be reasonably even across all the patients/families surveyed, and those with schizophrenic-like disorders were few in number. However, the strongly positive response among the half who returned questionnaires was from the patients' parents, as far as could be judged from the form and content of the answers. We were unable to say how many if any non-respondents failed to respond because the task had been left to the patient, or if it represented a view about the letters, or whether it said something about teenagers or the family dynamic. This highlights the problems of using limited and confidential questionnaires and emphasising their confidentiality, but it also draws attention to another problem: if a family is seen, and in child and adolescent psychiatry this is almost always with a single 'identified patient', who should be invited to complete the questionnaire? Should everyone who attended respond individually? Or should a consensus be invited?

The high level of response from family doctors was encouraging, and their generally very positive reactions interesting; in particular I had perhaps not expected such general emphasis on trust and openness among the general comments. If anything, it made me particularly thoughtful about what the small number who had urged caution had said, especially as two had referred specifically to not passing on sensitive information that had come from the family doctor. This might be the doctor's own views or a comment passed on from someone else, who also might not expect his or her thoughts to appear in due course in a letter back to the family. Throughout this book I hope I have emphasised sufficiently that letters should be only about what emerged in a session; these comments are additional reminders to be extra careful that such 'hearsay' information that comes into a session doesn't leak into the letter.

Psychiatrists, especially child and adolescent psychiatrists, receive referrals from a wide range of other workers, and I would expect different professional groups to respond differently.

In drawing conclusions about this study, it is worth bearing in mind the words of caution in the reviews by Williams (1994) and Thomas (1998) that respondents in surveys of patients' 'satisfaction' might in any case be generally inclined to reply positively, particularly if they have reasonably positive feelings about the staff whom they saw. In fact they are likely to have rather more complex ideas and feelings about the matters being surveyed than simple responses like 'helpful' and 'unhelpful' can convey. Williams points out that in recent years 'consumer satisfaction' has gained ground in health services as a measure of quality, and that results based on this may be misleading. In many ways this study of families' responses to letters was closer to a consumer survey than a detailed examination of thoughts and feelings about the letters, and the outcome should be interpreted in this light.

My first main conclusion, and despite the generally positive response we received, is uncertainty about what the adolescents and other non-respondents felt about the letters. All we can say is that at least half of the parents found the letters helpful. Second, despite the general view among our small sample of family doctors that their permission need not be sought to send patients copies of the consultant's letter, I would rather continue to seek their permission and, unless other data came along, this is the advice I would give about such letters.

Finally, I am reminded about the complexity of trying to conduct even a modest survey of this sort. Even the question of to whom to address the questionnaires, and different responses from different members of the family, raises methodological problems. An alternative might be to set aside some time at the point of discharge to discuss key letters, perhaps partly on a semi-structured basis. This could fit in with a concluding review not only of progress in general but of the patient's and family's experience of treatment.

Chapter 10

Conclusions

Information, authority and the letter

In the negotiated misunderstanding that is psychotherapy and much of treatment generally, a letter – something in writing – provides a fixed point. It is a statement, and, like other formal statements such as a motto, poem or symbol, it has an authority of its own. A conversation is a process, and is fluid. The letter holds the process still, freezing it. Reader and writer can see where the process seems to have got to at that point, and where it is leading so far. They have the chance to see if they are in agreement.

One of the values of a letter is that it should be informative, and being a written document it can be re-read and thought about. The possession of information is a considerable part of authority. Having the letter gives the patient the authority of knowledge and understanding, almost as if he or she had read a book or attended a course on the subject. The letter will not be comprehensive, but then nor is every book or course absorbed or even properly understood. I think a letter might be; at least, it is a hypothesis.

The letter is something from the writer to the recipient about themselves and about the problem, and one which can be a distillation of what the specialist knows and thinks he understands about the problem and the person. Recipients can use, discard, question, clarify or challenge it as they wish. It seems to me that the distribution of authority in this situation is not the same as the scene in the consulting room, where the expert explains the situation to the client. With the letter, the expert is more vulnerable. He or she makes it clear, or not. A letter generates feelings but can be read all over again. That which seemed initially clear or ambiguous can be reconsidered and found to be the opposite. A conversation generates feelings but there is a finality about the session; the clinician writes in the notes something about the explanation of the problem, the treatment or the prognosis. A videotape might show the expert explaining things patiently and the patient listening attentively, perhaps nodding, perhaps apparently agreeing that there are no questions to ask. But the patient might still go away puzzled, with questions unasked, some of them hard to put into words.

Letters in the context of clinical communication

There is an image of the doctor at the bedside which has become almost archetypal. The physician is doing nothing noticeable except being there, a grave and sympathetic presence. Indeed, in the period from which this picture dates, the imagined Golden Age of medicine, there was little he could do to change the course of events, a fact which appears to have diminished his authority remarkably little. Now that the technical possibilities of medical science are infinitely greater, medical authority is assailed on every side, and thus the picture seems to have changed completely: more technical expertise, more possibilities, practical and ethical, more discontent and distrust. And yet in a final twist medicine *still* remains obstinately at the top of the lists of most highly esteemed professions. Perhaps it is a good example of fuzzy logic, that *some* doctors are still supposedly wonderful, competent or both, that even their sternest critics tend to seek their help in the end, that with an infinity of needs, views and individuals the right person and problem can still click on to the right doctor, so the system and the status is kept conveniently afloat. That is a nod in the direction of one side of the brain, while the other side knows that it is only an attempt to rationalise magic. The archetypal doctor is like the archetypal magician, allowed, indeed needed, to take charge of that which is threatening but beyond our control, like madness and death. *Someone* has to stand for the notion that everything possible is being done. So even now, with the technical possibilities and public information vast and still accelerating, we need the role, and a person to take it, of the figure who will control the situation; even if that figure says something like 'Why don't *you* control it?', as surgeon, obstetrician or psychiatrist might, because the invitation can apply as much to holding the baby or taking a decision about genetics as to taking responsibility in a difficult and ambiguous psychological situation. Thus *permission* is still as important as consent.

I think this broad grey area around the archetypal doctor–patient relationship, particularly to do with authority, pervades most if not all other therapist relationships too, and if many sorts of psychotherapist spend time undoing assumptions of authority in their training and work, that only confirms the point. Communication, including written communication, must take account of the clinician's real or imagined authority.

There are many reasons for misunderstanding, including the patient's feelings and the clinician's feelings getting in the way of clear communication, and infinite varieties of collusion; for example, the patient who wants to be reassured and the doctor who wants to reassure, or the unspoken agreement not to talk about something. There is a very large literature on these aspects of the professional–client relationship, and it would be too large a diversion to review it here, but Angold (1994), Balint (1957), Bennet (1979, 1987), Byrne and Long (1976), Fraser (1976), Jenkins (1994), Joyce (1964) and Menzies (1970) offer some ways in, and elsewhere I have tried to view the problem via the issue of the nature of informed consent, since looking at dilemmas of authority and consent through the binocular vision of this dual concept (thus, what information is needed for properly informed consent?)

provides some clues to the way through a legal and ethical maze that is inevitably going to become increasingly complex (Steinberg, 1992a).

Let us accept that the doctor–patient relationship is more complex than meets the eye, that this can get in the way of understanding, decision-making and consent, and that recording something on paper makes a modest, pragmatic contribution to helping with the problem by putting some of the interaction literally on hold.

Paradox: an attempt to be clear about ambiguity

The use of paradox in therapy or in letters troubles me a little. It occupies an odd place in communication in that it can be manipulative and honest at the same time. This probably says something about the normal rules of communication. A simple example of a paradoxical instruction, or injunction, would be to advise the pathologically over-protective parent of an adolescent not to leave his side for an instant; that the parent should give up his or her job and get someone else to undertake social commitments and domestic chores, so that the logic of the parental position is taken to its limit. The young person's parent sees, or feels, the unreasonableness of attempting this, directly or indirectly resists it, and the anomalous position of over-protectiveness, with the fixity that goes with psychoneurosis, is destabilised.

Another example would be to point out to an anxious or depressed person that in the circumstances being described he or she seems not to be anxious or sad *enough*. In a situation where this type of intervention might help, a significant part of the patient's problems with feelings might seem to be preventing their expression and undermining treatment at the same time; thus instead of really accepting and working with bad feelings, they are siphoned off into the less productive task of trying to encourage unfeeling and uncomprehending therapists to ever greater efforts. The therapeutic response, that the patient might well need to be more distressed, not less, may be precisely right in terms of the psychopathology of the problem and the best way of proceeding in therapy, yet it is also paradoxical.

A similar approach was used in the cases of the young patients disabled, it seemed, by a behavioural response to distress rather than to physical illness (Letters 23 and 24 are examples of the cases, not of paradox); in one case physical investigations continued to a limited degree, in the other it was advised that they cease, but in both cases the child and family were told that as a psychiatric team we weren't the experts in pursuing complex neurological and neurobiochemical investigations (that had been the special expertise of the referrers), in which areas we had little to offer compared with the experts, that we could do little but accept the possibility of incurable illness, but fortunately we *were* confident about the team's rehabilitative skills with young people who suffered chronic disability. Was this paradoxical, or true? True, I think, in terms of such factual data as there was, yet it would be a paradoxical reply to a question (as if from a lawyer) like 'Can you cure this disease? Yes or no?'

All this is by way of acknowledging the possible rationale and integrity of the use of paradox. The therapist appears to be deliberately misunderstanding the patient's message; in fact he or she is focusing on one of a number of messages, the one which the therapist hopes will lead out of the tangle of mixed and contradictory messages that make up neuroses. In this sense the use of paradox is rather like the use of interpretation; indeed it is based on interpretation, and like interpretation it should be used within the context of the therapeutic relationship. Outside that relationship the casual use of paradox and interpretations is facile and inappropriate, and since one of the problems of letters is that one cannot know in what frame of mind they will be read or reread, interpretations and paradoxes should not be used in them. On the other hand a letter could refer to a discussion that took place in the consulting room and which may have been paradoxical or interpretive.

There is a different sort of ambiguity in the letter which is vague in the sense of being open-ended. Letters may very appropriately state or imply uncertainty, where uncertainty is the case: 'I don't know whether you want another appointment', or 'perhaps we should just see how it goes' put not only the decision but the decision about *making* a decision into the recipient's court, which can be perfectly appropriate. Ambiguity in this sense can contribute to a letter being consultative, because consultation too is not only about how to proceed but about who is to decide how to proceed: not necessarily the clinician.

Paradox is about the therapist's plans; ambiguity is about the therapist's questions.

The material letter

Why send a letter? Why not a fax or e-mail? Leaving aside the extra problems of confidentiality perhaps you could, and I hope what is discussed in this book will be helpful there too. But I think there is something more personal in the written, signed letter on paper, folded and placed in an envelope and which can be picked up, held, read, shared, torn up, screwed up, burned or otherwise discarded by the recipient. It could be kept and treasured, or as something to be held against the writer.

It's good, of course, if it's signed. I think it's wonderful if it is signed in ink, but that's a personal quirk. A signature typed in the same typography of the letter is preferable to a bogus signature in fancy type. I would prefer a rubber stamp. Sometimes, with the letter's dictator and its typist working to different schedules and in different places a 'p.p.' is resorted to. It is generally taken to mean *per pro*, 'for and on behalf of', and thus it seems perfectly logical for a secretary to put his or her name in front of the absentee: thus S. Fanny Adams p.p. Magnus B. Manifold. I only mention a contrary view (that p.p. should go before the secretary's name) for historical interest, because I have been assured by more than one distinguished archivist that what p.p. really stands for is *per proxime*, that is 'by one authorised as nearest', indeed as his or her proxy; hence Magnus B. Manifold p.p. S. Fanny Adams makes sense.

Does everyone else know that c.c. means 'carbon copy'? I didn't.

In letters, we say things that may be uncharacteristic of both the writer and reader; we address each other as Dear, which is rather nice; we say Yours sincerely if we address someone by name (Yours faithfully, of course, if we don't); we may say Yours, mysteriously and ambiguously if feeling really friendly. Strong men like to say Yours ever. Such words reflect another sort of world, and it is not surprising that it is beginning to be nibbled away at the edges through various forms of words that I will not encourage by reproducing here. But I would be pleasantly surprised if Dear is still in general use this time next century.

A nicety I have observed in letters is the transition between, for example, Dear Professor Sir Alfred Hart Biggs and Dear Alf. People who communicate by correspondence rather than in person are often not as confident as junk mail companies about going straight into first name terms, and the writer may dictate Dear Professor, etc. and then, on signing the letter, draw a neat line through the extended name and substitute Dear Alf, as if in an inspired afterthought. Actually I find it rather corny, but the strategy does have a certain stuffy charm.

More charmingly old-fashioned is 'Dear Bessy, if I may', though this is now quite rare. I also believe that if the letter writer doesn't indicate his or her title (e.g. Mr, Mrs, Miss, Ms) it can be taken that it doesn't matter how you reply; similarly, when even the name is omitted, illegible or untyped. You could glue the offending ending to the front of the reply envelope.

In a small way a letter is a gift or a token, and some letters in some situations may have some of the magical qualities of the prescription, which traditionally begins, as mentioned earlier (p.3), with the magic symbol Rx. This is often printed on the form to save the magician the trouble, along with various official questions and regulations. I don't want to make too much of this, but I don't think we should ignore it completely.

Finally, it can be initially frustrating in an organisation, though ultimately rewarding, to show an interest in the design of letterheads and hospital and clinic logos, and indeed in all the printed literature that represents your own and your colleagues' work. It is astonishing how poor they can be, considering the good designs that are available. Symbols are important.

Therapeutic communication and the internet

I have not discussed the use of the telephone in therapy and follow-up because the spoken word, even on the phone, is so close to the real live therapeutic relationship, while this book is about the written word as complementing it. However, tele-communications have dramatically caught up with the written word, and the use of electronic means of written communication in counselling and psychotherapy seems to be with us to stay. A growing literature has reviewed the use of e-mail in therapy (Murphy and Mitchell, 1998), questioned how various definitions of intimacy apply within electronic communication (Robson and Robson, 1998), looked at the ethical issues in counselling on the world wide web with particular reference to confidentiality, counsellor qualities and skills and the validity of the information exchanged (Bloom, 1998), and explored the use of the internet to involve family members in joint work when they are geographically separated (e.g. Gale *et al.*,

1995). While this literature is largely concerned with therapy *primarily* by electronic communication, King *et al.* (1998) extend their discussion to the use of e-mail as a supplement to therapy.

Authority, consultation and the letter

There are many different sorts of authority. There is the authority of hard facts, or at least of facts which are on fairly firm ground in the light of what we know so far: most scientists acknowledge the teaching of Popper and others that all scientific knowledge is provisional (e.g. O'Hear, 1980). There is also the authority of experience, integrity and skill, and there ought to be enough in place in the referral process, and by way of information and openness generally, for the client to know what any specialist has to offer in these respects. All of this should help patients and clients use their own natural and legal authority to exercise choice to the full. This is where the consultative approach (pp. 11–13; 84) is helpful, because it is one way of sorting out by mutual agreement that which the expert contributes to the therapeutic work and that which, as mentioned above, the client contributes, in a process which allows and underpins properly informed consent.

Consultation helps distribute authority helpfully between the technical capability of the clinician (including the clinician's responsibility as teacher) and the authority of the patient as the owner of and expert on the problem (including the patient's responsibility to learn). In fact something along these lines happens when people discuss plans with builders, electricians and architects, but in the therapeutic relationship understanding and decision-making can become muddled and mislaid. Even lawyers, practitioners of that much maligned profession, operate by telling their clientele about the law, helping *them* decide how to proceed, and then speaking on their behalf as best they can. For all the practical and historical hitches and glitches between lawyers and their clients, it's a good professional model, that of the *advocate*, who gives voice to the client's predicament and the possible remedies.

The model letter, with its many necessary variations, should serve this sort of function. It should literally address those involved, identify the issues (mentioning who has put what on the agenda), add the writer's suggestions about what to make of it and how to proceed, and in one way or another invite the recipients to give their comments. If a consultation is envisaged as a group of people working on a problem, the letter should be the equivalent of a provisional agenda and a rough outline indicating some of the headings for the minutes. If the therapeutic process is perceived in terms of roles and drama, the letter is like a draft script or 'treatment' inviting the comments of the other participants.

The anatomy of the letter: a summary

- There should be a correct and complete address, one that works in getting the letter to precisely the right individual or group and addresses them individually in a way which works with the therapeutic relationship and the therapeutic task. *Always* remember that a letter in the post is bound to be that much less secure than notes in a filing cabinet. In fact, an office intruder may well come across or hack into private information which seems of no special interest, while the 'other person' in a family or locality who sees a letter which they shouldn't may be close enough to the recipient for it to matter.

- There should be indications of sensitive, thoughtful practice: reasonable paper and printing, correct spelling and grammar, and the proper respect and courtesies. Courtesies aren't trivia. They enable the smaller social processes and make the larger ones feasible; thus they will make it more likely that a letter is read, and make it at least possible that painful, difficult or merely tedious matters are engaged with.

- The letter should convey with clarity what the writer means, unless the intention is to be ambiguous, which should be done with care and with a clear reason (pp. 2; 116–117). Mystification, psychodynamic interpretation and the use of paradox should be avoided *de novo* in a letter, but if interpretation or paradox has been used in a session, and thus is part of therapy, I think it is reasonable for the theme to be pursued.

- Feelings, and therefore new material, should be handled with care. As mentioned on page 9, letters are a useful form of displacement; they represent ways of using detachment, distancing and objectivity in therapy and as such have their limitations as well as their uses.

- There should be an indication of what seems to the writer to constitute the facts of the matter, that is, the size and shape of the problem and the options about how to proceed as the writer sees it. The facts may be about the clinical and social realities of a situation, including the feasible options; or they may be in terms of what good practice would suggest, or what is indicated by evidence-based treatment; or it will often be simply descriptive – the child who will not go to school, the situation or symptom that is resisting change.

- Use what was in the session, and as far as possible what individuals said about themselves and those present. Take care with comments about those not present.

- The writer should give his or her views and advice.

- There should be the possibility, invitation and encouragement for the recipients to choose from options, bearing in mind that if this power is differential (for example, between adults and children) that too will be among the relevant facts.

- There should be some reference or guidelines to the structure and organisation of the work being undertaken; not only reminders of past or next appointments, if that happens to be appropriate, but also acknowledgement of the context in which the letter is being written. For example, that we (therapist and clientele) are stuck or in disagreement or have a decision to make or that all is going well, and so on.

- Take care with confidentiality. There are many different aspects of this, and I would advise looking up the various references to it in the index.

Much of the above will be extensively modified, perhaps only alluded to, or simply just thought about when deciding what to write. Some of it will be left out entirely. Like mammalian anatomy it is mostly all there, but may be adapted and modified for different purposes.

Taken overall, the letter should therefore provide the reader with a reasonably factual view of how things seem to the writer, but it should also invite or enable the recipient to join in; therefore it should also incorporate qualities that contribute to the atmosphere in which joint conclusion-reaching or decision-making is possible. It is hard to be precise about this, but the nuances of language can variously induce warmth, interest, friendliness, anxiety, sadness, confusion, paranoia and rage, and this affects both how the tasks indicated in the letter are handled, and the wider processes involved in therapy.

It is the something extra that is more difficult to define precisely, because it is an attempt to distil into writing the current work of the therapeutic relationship, as well as something of the atmosphere and setting of the consultation. There is a whole new area of work examining how clinics and similar settings can be positive, attractive, *aesthetic* environments which complement therapy and help recovery (e.g. Haldane and Loppert, 1999; Senior and Croall, 1993) in ways that go further than the aims and methods of the arts therapies. Reading and writing (by patients and by staff) is part of this work (e.g. Bolton, 1996; Jones, 1990), while Tonfoni (1994) has described writing and reading as a process and psychological and physical experience which places writing among the visual arts. The act of writing, the writing itself, and reading what is written, can go beyond (though never leave behind) the meanings in the words themselves, and like other arts can contribute to physical and emotional well-being, indeed to sanity, and complement treatment. Perhaps the letters we write can contribute to this. The reader will know by now whether this may be worthwhile, possible or even interesting.

Epilogue

Among a number of curious old books on my shelves are some elderly guides to the writing of letters, all very much in the Victorian and Edwardian tradition of self-improvement and, of course, the improvement of others. They make amusing reading: how to apply for a job, how to warn an unsuitable man away from your daughter, how to seek the repayment of a debt (or seek credit) and how to turn down an unwelcome suitor. They sometimes end with earnest and glorious flourishes like

'With Kind Remembrances,
Believe Me, Dear Madam,
I Remain, and Am,
Yours Very Sincerely',

etc. The author occasionally hides modestly behind some such title as 'A member of the Aristocracy'.

I mention all this largely for amusement, partly to acknowledge these honourable past efforts in public instruction, but also to reiterate that this really hasn't been intended as a 'how to' book. I suppose it has struck me, looking back through the pages, that it might resemble one. Rather, I have tried to illustrate the sort of dialogue which writers of such letters might have with themselves in trying to find the best words to capture on paper significant moments in their work.

I am,
Yours, etc.

References

Albert, T. (1991) Undervalued skill of letter writing in general practice. *Pulse*, 28: 30–31.

Angold, A. (1994) Clinical interviewing with children and adolescents, in M. Rutter, E. Taylor and L. Hersov (eds) *Child and Adolescent Psychiatry: Modern Approaches*. Oxford: Blackwell Science.

Asch, R., Price, J.S. and Hawks, G. (1991) Psychiatric out-patients' reactions to summary letters of their consultations. *British Journal of Medical Psychology*, 64: 3–9.

Ayalon, O. (1990) *Crisis and Coping with Suicide and Bereavement*. Haifa: Nord Publications.

Balint, M. (1957) *The Doctor, his Patient and the Illness*. London: Pitman.

Bateson, G. (1972) *Steps to an Ecology of Mind*. New York: Ballantyne Books.

Bateson, G. (1979) *Mind and Nature: A Necessary Unity*. New York: Dutton.

Bennet, G. (1979) *Patients and Their Doctors*. London : Bailliere Tindall.

Bennet, G. (1987) *The Wound and the Doctor*. London: Secker and Warburg.

Berger, P. and Luckmann, T. (1967) *The Social Construction of Reality: A Treatise in the Sociology of Knowledge*. Harmondsworth: Penguin.

Bernadt, M., Gunning, L. and Questedt, M. (1991) Patients' access to their own psychiatric records. *British Medical Journal*, 303: 967.

Bettelheim, B. (1976) *The Uses of Enchantment: The Meaning and Importance of Fairy Tales*. London: Thames and Hudson.

Black, D., Wolkind, S. and Hendriks, J.H. (1998) *Child Psychiatry and the Law*, 3rd edn. London: Gaskell.

Bloom, J.W. (1998) The ethical practice of web counseling. *British Journal of Guidance and Counselling*, 26(1): 53–59.

Bolton, D. and Hill, J. (1996) *Mind, Meaning and Mental Disorder: The Nature of Causal Explanation in Psychology and Psychiatry*. Oxford: Oxford University Press.

Bolton, G. (1996) The process of writing gets me in touch. *Artery, The Journal of Arts for Health*, 14: 15–16.

Brahams, D. (1994) Right of access to medical records. *Lancet*, 344: 743.

Brown, D. and Pedder, J. (1979) *Introduction to Psychotherapy*. London: Tavistock.

Butler, R.E. and Nicholls, D.E. (1993) The Access to Health Records Act: what difference does it make? *Psychiatric Bulletin*, 17: 204–206.

Byrne, P.S. and Long, B.E.L. (1976) *Doctors Talking to Patients: A Study of the Verbal Behaviour of General Practitioners Consulting in their Surgeries*. London: Her Majesty's Stationery Office.

Campbell, J. (1973) *The Masks of God, Volume 4 Creative Mythology*. London: Souvenir Press.

Caplan, G. (1970) *The Theory and Practice of Mental Health Consultation*. London: Tavistock.

Dare, C. (1985) Family therapy, in M. Rutter and L. Hersov (eds) *Child and Adolescent Psychiatry: Modern Approaches*, 3rd edn. Oxford: Blackwell Scientific Publications.

Dwivedi, K.N. and Gardner, D. (1997) Theoretical perspectives and clinical approaches, in K.N. Dwivedi (ed.) *The Therapeutic Use of Stories*. London: Routledge.

Eaden, J.A., Ward, B. and Smith, H. (1998) Are we telling patients enough? A pilot study to assess patient information needs in a gastroenterology out-patient department. *European Journal of Gastroenterology*, 10: 63–67.

Eisenberg, L. (1975) The ethics of intervention: acting amidst ambiguity. *Journal of Child Psychology and Psychiatry*, 16: 93–104.

Ellis, C. (1989) Epistotherapy. *British Medical Journal*, 299: 1230.

Foucault, M. (1980) *Power/Knowledge: Selected Interviews and Other Writings*. New York: Pantheon.

Frank, A.W. (1993) The rhetoric of self-change: illness experience as narrative. *The Sociological Quarterly*, 34: 39–52.

Fraser, C. (1976) An analysis of face-to-face communication, in A.E. Bennett (ed.) *Communication Between Doctors and Patients*. Oxford: Oxford University Press.

Gale, J., Dotson, D., Huber, M. and Young, K. (1995) A new technology for teaching/learning. *Marital and Family Therapy*, 21: 183–191.

Gass, W.H. (1972) *Fiction and the Figures of Life*. New York: Vintage.

Gauthier, J. (1999) Writing to families. *Psychiatric Bulletin*, 23: 387–389.

Goldberg, D. (1996) 'Emplotment: Letters in Child Psychiatry', paper given at meeting of the Regional Association of Child and Adolescent Psychiatrists, Ticehurst House Hospital. (Unpublished).

Gorell Barnes, G. (1985) Systems theory and family theory, in M. Rutter and L. Hersov (eds) *Child and Adolescent Psychiatry: Modern Approaches*. Oxford: Blackwell Scientific Publications.

Gorell Barnes, G. (1994) Family therapy, in M. Rutter, E. Taylor and L. Hersov (eds) *Child and Adolescent Psychiatry: Modern Approaches*, 3rd edn. Oxford: Blackwell Scientific Publications.

Haldane, D. and Loppert, S. (1999) *The Arts in Health Care*. London: King's Fund Publishing.

Hoffman, L. (1990) Constructing realities: an art of lenses. *Family Process*, 29: 1–12.

Holmes, J. (1994) *John Bowlby and Attachment Theory*. London: Routledge.

Jenkins, H. (1994) Family interviewing: aspects of theory and practice, in M. Rutter, E. Taylor and L. Hersov (eds) *Child and Adolescent Psychiatry: Modern Approaches*. Oxford: Blackwell Science.

Jones, A.H. (1990) Literature and medicine: traditions and innovations, in C. Clarke and F. Aycock (eds) *The Body and the Text*. Texas: Texas Tech University Press.

Joyce, C.R.B. (1964) What does the doctor let the patient tell him? *Journal of Psychosomatic Research*, 8: 343–352.

King, S.A., Engi, S. and Poulos, S.T. (1998) Using the internet to assist family therapy. *British Journal of Guidance and Counselling*, 26(1): 43–52.

L'Abate, L. and Platzman, K. (1991) The practice of programmed writing (PW) in therapy and prevention with families. *American Journal of Family Therapy*, 19: 99–109.

Laing, R.D. (1970) *Knots*. Harmondsworth: Penguin.

Leff, J.P., Kuipers, L., Berkowitz, R. and Sturgeon, D. (1985) A controlled trial of inter-vention in the families of schizophrenic patients: a two-year follow up. *British Journal of Psychiatry*, 146: 594–600.

McLaren, P. (1991) The right to know: patients' records should be understandable by patients, too. *British Medical Journal*, 303: 937–938.

Mattingly, C. (1994) The concept of therapeutic 'emplotment'. *Social Science and Medicine*, 38(6): 811–822.

Menzies, I. (1970) *The Functioning of Social Systems as a Defence Against Anxiety*. London: Tavistock Institute of Human Relations, Pamphlet No. 3.

Minuchin, S., Rosman, B.L. and Baker, L. (1980) *Psychosomatic Families: Anorexia Nervosa in Context*. Cambridge, MA: Harvard University Press.

Murphy, L.J. and Mitchell, D.L. (1998) When writing helps to heal: e-mail as therapy. *British Journal of Guidance and Counselling*, 26(1): 21–32.

Nell, V. (1988) *Lost in a Book*. New Haven, CT: Yale University Press.

O'Hear, A. (1980) *Karl Popper*. London: Routledge & Kegan Paul.

Orwell, G. (1949) *Nineteen Eighty-four*. London: Secher and Warburg.

Parrott, J., Strathede, G. and Brown, P. (1988) Patient access to psychiatric records: the patient's view. *Journal of the Royal Society of Medicine*, 81: 520–522.

Penn, P. and Frankfurt, M. (1994) Creating a participant text: writing, multiple voices, narrative multiplicity. *Family Process*, 33: 217–231.

Pierides, M. (1999) Writing to patients. *Psychiatric Bulletin*, 23: 385–386.

Roberts, G. and Holmes, J. (eds) (1999) *Healing Stories: Narrative in Psychiatry and Psychotherapy*. Oxford: Oxford University Press.

Robson, D. and Robson, M. (1998) Intimacy and computer communication. *British Journal of Guidance and Counselling*, 26(1): 33–41.

Rogers, C.R. (1951) *Client-centered Therapy*. Boston, MA: Houghton Mifflin Co.

Ryle, A. (1982) *Psychotherapy: A Cognitive Integration of Theory and Practice*. London: Academic Press.

Senior, P. and Croall, J. (1993) *Helping to Heal: The Arts in Health Care*. London: Calouste Gulbenkian Foundation.

Shah, P.J. and Pullen, I. (1995) The impact of a hospital audit on psychiatrists' letters to general practitioners. *Psychiatric Bulletin*, 19: 544–547.

Shiryon, M. (1978) Literatherapy: theory and application, in R.J. Rubin (ed.) *Bibliotherapy Sourcebook*. New York: Oryx Press.

Skynner, A.C.R. (1975) The large group in training, in L. Kreeger (ed.) *The Large Group: Dynamics and Therapy*. London: Constable.

Sloman, L. and Pipitone, J. (1991) Letter writing in family therapy. *American Journal of Family Therapy*, 19: 77–82.

Steinberg, D. (1981) *Using Child Psychiatry: The Functions and Operations of a Specialty*. London: Hodder and Stoughton.

Steinberg, D. (1983) *The Clinical Psychiatry of Adolescence. Clinical Work from a Social and Developmental Perspective*. Chichester, Sussex: John Wiley.

Steinberg, D. (ed.) (1986) *The Adolescent Unit: Work and Teamwork in Adolescent Psychiatry*. Chichester, Sussex: John Wiley.

Steinberg, D. (1987) *Basic Adolescent Psychiatry*. Oxford: Blackwell Science.

Steinberg, D. (1989) *Interprofessional Consultation: Innovation and Imagination in Working Relationships*. Oxford: Blackwell Science.

Steinberg, D. (1992a) Informed consent: consultation as a basis for collaboration between disciplines and between professionals and their patients. *Journal of Interprofessional Care*, 61: 43–48.

Steinberg, D. (1992b) Consultative work in child and adolescent psychiatry. *Archives of Disease in Childhood*, 67: 1302–1305.

Steinberg, D. (1993) Consultative work in child and adolescent psychiatry, in M.E. Garralda (ed.) *Managing Children with Psychiatric Problems*. London: BMJ Publishing Group.

Steinberg, D. (1999) Interprofessional consultation and creative approaches in therapeutic work across cultures, in J. Kareem and R. Littlewood (eds) *Intercultural Therapy*, 2nd edn. Oxford: Blackwell Science.

Steinberg, D. (2000) The psychiatrist as consultant to schools and colleges, in M.G. Gelder, J. Lopez-Ibor and N.C. Andreasan (eds) *The New Oxford Textbook of Psychiatry*. Oxford: Oxford University Press.

Steinberg, D. (in press) Art and Consciousness.

Stubbs, M. (1980) *Language and Literacy: The Socialinguistics of Reading and Writing*. London: Routledge and Kegan Paul.

Swanson, J.M., Sergeant, J.A., Taylor, E., Sonuga-Barke, E.J.S., Jensen, P.S. and Cantwell, D.P. (1998) Attention-deficit hyperactivity disorder and hyperkinetic disorder. *Lancet*, 351: 429–432.

Thomas, P. (1998) Writing letters to patients. *Psychiatric Bulletin*, 22: 542–545.

Tonfoni, G. (1994) *Writing as a Visual Art*. Oxford: Intellect Books.

Tufnell, G., Cottrell, D. and Georgiades, D. (1996) 'Good practice' for expert witnesses. *Clinical Child Psychology and Psychiatry*, 1(3): 365–383.

Tyrer, P. and Steinberg, D. (1998) *Models for Mental Disorder: Conceptual Models in Psychiatry*, 3rd edn. Chichester, Sussex: John Wiley.

Von Bertalanffy, L. (1968) *General Systems Theory*. New York: George Brazillier.

White, M. and Epston, D. (1990) *Narrative Means to Therapeutic Ends*. London: W.W. Norton.

Williams, B. (1994) Patient satisfaction: a valid concept? *Social Science and Medicine*, 38: 509–516.

Winnicott, D.W. (1972) *The Maturational Process and the Facilitating Environment*. London: The Hogarth Press.

Young, J.W. (1991) *Totalitarian Language: Orwell's Newspeak and its Nazi and Communist Antecedents*. Charlottesville: University of Virginia Press.

General index

Clinical index

aetiology 87, 102
age of consent, issues concerning 28, 29, 64, 89
alcohol misuse 32, 66, 72, 89
anger 38, 42, 45, 52, 54, 69, 73
anorexia nervosa 103
anxiety, parental 29, 38
anxiety state 85, 86, 96
arts, in healthcare 121
Asperger's syndrome *see* autistic spectrum disorder
attention deficit hyperactivity disorder (ADHD) 61, 62
authority, family problems with 25, 52
authority, in therapy 28, 65, 69, 70, 74; *see also* General index
autism *see* autistic spectrum disorder
autistic spectrum disorder 34, 37, 95

bed wetting *see* enuresis
behaviour problems 30, 61, 62, 79
behaviour therapy 13, 51, 59
bell and pad (night alarm) 57, 58, 59, 72
bereavement 6; *see also* grief; loss
body language 44
boundaries; and family problems with 2, 68, 80; *see also* illness behaviour
boredom 56, 57
bullying, at school 42, 44, 45

chaos and anomaly, in family 20, 25, 32
chronic problems, developmental 34ff., 94ff., 97, 116
cognitive analytic therapy, and letters 6, 110
compulsory treatment 29, 90
conduct disorder *see* behaviour problems

countertransference 21

death 45, 49, 50
delinquency 30, 32, 62
depression: in adolescents 25, 48, 57, 75, 96; *see also* manic depression; in parents 48ff.
developmental problems 37, 39, 41, 75, 77, 79
diagnosis vs. description 39, 42
disability 39
drug misuse 32, 66, 87, 88, 89
drug therapy *see* medication

education *see* school and college, training
encopresis 73, 74
enuresis 57, 59, 60, 73

family therapy, family work 13, 37, 40, 44, 46, 47, 48, 63, 65, 85, 90

grief, parental and loss 41, 42

handicap *see* disability
healing, spiritual 92–94
hyperactivity *see* attention deficit hyperactivity disorder (ADHD)
hysteria *see* illness behaviour

illness behaviour 76ff., 78
independence, issues of 39, 89
insomnia 86
investigations, medical 35, 40
interpretation 117, 120
intrusiveness, parental 69, 70, 80, 81

learning disorder 78